Praise for *High Steaks*

Although all life is exquisitely interconnected by air, water and soil, we have shattered that world through the way we perceive it in bits and pieces, so we fail to recognize that our lifestyle has repercussions that reverberate through the biosphere. Industrial agriculture creates food by converting the energy in oil rather than directly from sunlight into plants. Eleanor Boyle's timely book, *High Steaks*, reconnects our fragmented view to reveal the ecological, social, health and economic costs of a diet rich in meat. This is a vital book for all concerned about the perilous state of our planet and anxious for ways to live that are healthy for ourselves and the biosphere.

— David Suzuki, scientist, environmentalist and author

This is a very important book — it addresses a key component of our climate troubles, and it does it by addressing people where they actually are, and offering some realistic, attractive, and compelling options for changing deep-rooted habits.

— Bill McKibben, author
Eaarth: Making a Life on a Tough New Planet

The list of mainstream meat production's negative impacts is long: health, climate change, land use, feedstock, water, pharmaceutical misuse, biodiversity. A better course can and is being charted. This must engage all of us.

— Tim Lang, Professor of Food Policy,
City University London

In some future century, humanity will either become comfortable with eating meat or will quit eating meat. For now, as Eleanor Boyle explains in her well-researched and well-written book, our individual health and the sustainability of our society depend on rejecting industrial agriculture, which includes eating less meat. Boyle gives us dozens of good reasons to eat more responsibly and sustainably.

— John Ikerd, Author, Speaker, and
Professor Emeritus of Agricultural Economics,
University of Missouri, Columbia.

For years we have been encouraged to eat more meat than what is good for us and the planet. Eleanor Boyle presents reasonable and compelling arguments for moving meat from the centre of our plates to the side. Whether you care about your family's health, our environment, how farm animals are treated or all of the above, this book is an essential read. This isn't another doom and gloom book. Instead it shows how we can all be part of the solution and achieve a more humane and sustainable food system. After reading Eleanor Boyle's book, it is hard to imagine who wouldn't support a food system that is healthier for society, gentler on the planet and kinder to animals. She presents reasonable and compelling evidence to demonstrate that our current meat consumption levels are not sustainable as well as recipes for change. By changing our food policies and a few meals a week, we can all be part of the solution and improve our health, the environment and animal welfare.

— Melissa Matlow, Campaigns Manager,
Humane and Sustainable Agriculture
World Society for the Protection of Animals (WSPA) — Canada

A thorough, encompassing, and refreshingly balanced analysis of what it means to eat meat. The author provides compelling evidence that meat, and specifically that which evolves from high density confinement feeding systems, affects the health and welfare of people, communities, livestock and the broader environment. Rigorous citation of recent refereed literature makes this a must-read text for those seeking the latest, scientific understanding of many contentious issues. Articulate, comfortable, and readable prose ensures that the critical content of this book is accessible to a wide range of readers.

— E. Ann Clark, Associate Professor (retired)
Plant Agriculture, University of Guelph

HIGH STEAKS

WHY AND HOW TO EAT LESS MEAT

Eleanor Boyle

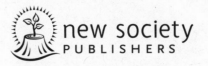
new society
PUBLISHERS

Cover design by Diane McIntosh.
Background image, © iStock (bopshops); Illustration © iStock (Oehoeboero)
Printed in Canada by Friesens. First printing July 2012.

New Society Publishers acknowledges the support of the Government of Canada through the Book Publishing Industry Development Program (BPIDP) for our publishing activities.

Paperback ISBN: 978-0-86571-713-8   eISBN: 978-1-55092-499-2

Inquiries regarding requests to reprint all or part of *High Steaks* should be addressed to New Society Publishers at the address below.

To order directly from the publishers, please call toll-free (North America) 1-800-567-6772, or order online at www.newsociety.com

Any other inquiries can be directed by mail to:

New Society Publishers
P.O. Box 189, Gabriola Island, BC V0R 1X0, Canada
(250) 247-9737

LIBRARY AND ARCHIVES CANADA CATALOGUING IN PUBLICATION

Boyle, Eleanor, 1953–
High steaks : why and how to eat less meat / Eleanor Boyle.

Includes index.
ISBN 978-0-86571-713-8

1. Livestock — Ecology.   2. Animal industry — Environmental
aspects.   3. Animal culture.   4. Food of animal origin — Health
aspects.   5. Animals — Food.   I. Title.

SF140.E25B69 2012   338.1'76   C2012-903959-4

New Society Publishers' mission is to publish books that contribute in fundamental ways to building an ecologically sustainable and just society, and to do so with the least possible impact on the environment, in a manner that models this vision. We are committed to doing this not just through education, but through action. The interior pages of our bound books are printed on Forest Stewardship Council®-registered acid-free paper that is **100% post-consumer recycled** (100% old growth forest-free), processed chlorine free, and printed with vegetable-based, low-VOC inks, with covers produced using FSC®-registered stock. New Society also works to reduce its carbon footprint, and purchases carbon offsets based on an annual audit to ensure a carbon neutral footprint. For further information, or to browse our full list of books and purchase securely, visit our website at: www.newsociety.com

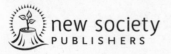

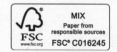

Contents

What's Wrong with Livestock? What's Wrong with Meat? •
Addressing Livestock and Meat Is Key to Food Security • We're
Capable of Eating Less and Better

PART 1: WHY? REASONS FOR EATING LESS MEAT

"…Now I Eat Meat Twice a Day" • We're Climbing the Food Chain
to Dangerous Heights • There's a Push for Mass Production and
Consumption • Excessive Supply Drives Excessive Demand

Meat Should Make Environmental Sense • Livestock Today Casts
a Long Shadow • It's Deforestation and It's Gas Production • In
Large Numbers, All Livestock Add to Climate Change • Wealthy
Countries need.to Lower Consumption

Activists Are Testing the Waters • Waste Is Not a Pretty Topic •
This Much Manure Isn't Fertilizer, It's Pollution • Water Around
the World Is Getting Wasted • Sufficient and Clean Water Should
Be Priorities

Moderation Is a Prescription for Health • Factory Farming Fuels
Animal-to-Human Diseases • Intensively Raised Livestock Get
Drugs • Antibiotics Are in a Class of Their Own • Lifestyle
Diseases Get a Hand from Too Much Meat • Healthy Solutions
Include Eating Less and Better

We Want Quality of Life • We Want Local Control • We Want

Food Systems to Strengthen Environmental Health • We Want
Food Systems to Reflect Our Values

PART 2: HOW? STRATEGIES FOR EATING LESS MEAT

It's Perfectly Acceptable to Ask People to Eat Less Meat •
Everyone Can Be Involved in This Project • Meat Can Be Made
More Sustainably • Social Systems Can Change. People Can
Change • How Much Less?

Take It from a Chef • We Can Be Personal Agents of Change •
We Can Develop New Attitudes and Strategies • We Can Be
Healthier by Eating Less Meat • We've Already Started This Project

Taxes Could Be on the Table • Meat Policy Should Be Central to
Food Policy • Policy Can Encourage Healthy Consumption •
Policy Can Improve Livestock Production • Two Key Strategy
Areas: Fewer Antibiotics and More Animal Welfare • Policy Needs
to Accommodate Farms Like Sap Bush Hollow • Solutions May
Require International Cooperation

Social Norms Can Shift • Meat-Eaters, Vegans, and Everyone
Else Can Be on the Same Team • Political Impediments Can Be
Addressed • Corporate Influence Can Be Questioned • We Can
Educate Ourselves About the Meat Problem • Citizens Can Prevail

The Meat Problem Is Amenable to Solutions • We Can Get
Inspired • High Steaks Is a Theme for Our Time

Acknowledgments

If it takes a village to raise a child, as the proverb says, it also takes a community to write a book. Thank you to researchers who first recognized and raised these issues and, during my research, to the many individuals who went out of their way to share their time and expertise. People who hosted me and hiked, drove, or flew me around their countryside included: in rural Ontario, Colleen Ross; in Lethbridge, Cheryl Bradley and Ann Baran and others; in Winnipeg, Glen Koroluk and Patrick Krawek; in North Carolina, Larry Baldwin, Rick Dove, Dennis Howard, and Joanne Somerday, John Klecker, Kelsey Hansen, Marty Lawrence, and Diane Baldwin. In southern Alberta, Francis and Bonnie Gardner and their daughter Sarah, and neighbor Gordon Cartwright, enriched my understanding. In upstate New York, thanks to Adele and Jim Hayes, and Shannon Hayes, for educating me and for hosting photographer Seth Joel.

People who consented to be interviewed included Hans Schreier, JoAnn Burkholder, Cathy Holtslander, Mike Williams, Mark Mattson, Don Webb, Elsie Herring, Naeema Muhammed, Gary Grant, Hannah Connor, E. Ann Clark, Fred Tait, Basia Romanowicz, and Conner Ingram. Eva Pip welcomed me to her lab and educated me on water quality. Rod MacRae provided me with historical context and an overview of policy. A warm thank you to chef Annie Somerville, who made time to take part and who inspired me with her excitement about good food. Industry experts who helped me understand producers' viewpoints included Mike Teillet, Dennis Treacy, Amy Richards, and Stewart Paulson.

Individuals who directly or indirectly shared ideas about food, environment, health, and/or animal protection include John Ikerd, Tara Garnett, Robert P. Martin, Laura Rogers, Kathy Phillips, Dawn Jackson Blatner, Steve Wing, Daniel Imhoff, Rajendra Pachauri, Barb Finley, Lisa Bechthold, Joyce Holmes, Elizabeth Brubaker, Leanne McConnachie, Wayne Roberts, Herb Barbolet, Nancy Callan, Brewster and Cathleen Kneen, and others. I heartily thank Joyce D'Silva who made time for meaningful discussions. Others who offered ideas include Julian Wake, Esther Chetner, and Peter Ladner. Supporting me with enthusiasm for the project were Melissa Matlow, Susan and Leonard Angel, Debbie Weinstein, and my family. People who read parts of the manuscript included Trevor Murdock, David Steele, Peter Fricker, Cathleen Boyle, Paul Turje, and Jon Festinger. I thank Henning Steinfeld and Pierre Gerber for meeting with me, and for helping spark a global discourse. I thank Anthony McMichael for offering me details on possible strategies for addressing the issues.

My appreciation to my mentors Tim Lang, David Barling and Martin Caraher at the Centre for Food Policy. They are world leaders in putting food policy on the public agenda, and studying with them was an honor.

In expressing appreciation to colleagues and supporters, I nevertheless take full responsibility for this book and its information and points of view.

I acknowledge the team at New Society Publishers for their support, professionalism, and flexibility, including Ingrid Witvoet, Heather Nicholas, Sara Reeves, Greg Green, Sue Custance, and EJ Hurst, and my skilled and collegial editor, Linda Glass. For research assistance, I thank David Cragg and Katherine Pybus, and for technical expertise, Seth Joel, web developer Matt Morrison, and Al Karim and his staff.

My gratitude to my parents who showed me how to eat modestly, healthfully, and minimizing waste. Finally, my love and appreciation to my husband, Harley Rothstein, who has been a constant source of motivation, support, and intellectual stimulation, and who has encouraged me to follow my passions.

Introduction:
The Steaks Are High

What's Wrong with Livestock? What's Wrong with Meat?

Pick up a menu from almost any restaurant and glance through the options. Chicken and pork, burgers and steak, ribs and wings, a couple of seafood items, and near the bottom one or two vegetarian options. Clearly, meat is what's to eat. The dietary dominance of flesh foods, especially from land animals, is such a strong norm that most of us don't question it. But the present status of meat as the main attraction at the center of the plate — across countries, cultures, and socio-economic groups — is unprecedented in human history. Never before on Earth has so much meat been produced and have so many people consumed so much.

An abundance of meat may sound like a solution, not a problem. All that sustenance, all those nutrients, all that delicious fare. But animal products today represent a crisis for the environment and public health. They also represent an opportunity if we, as consumers and communities, recognize and take the challenge on.

What's wrong with livestock? What's wrong with meat? In moderation, nothing — if you accept that humans have the moral right to use animals for food. Most people accept this — as I do — as long as we treat animals respectfully and maintain some reverence for taking their lives. For environmental or health reasons, there's nothing wrong with producing and consuming some flesh foods. Raising livestock allows us to employ animals and plants symbiotically in agriculture and ecosystems, and eating meat gives us nutrients and calories. But is it possible, as the

1

evidence increasingly suggests, that we're making and eating too much for the good of the planet and our personal and community well-being?

It's all about amounts. In times past, people generally ate animal products in small quantities or on special occasions. Besides, there were fewer of us. So our ancestors raised livestock by grazing a few cows and goats on marginal grasslands or integrating pigs and poultry into mixed farms where the animals ate scraps and provided fertilizer. But now that humans number seven billion, and with whole populations expecting bacon for breakfast, cold cuts for lunch, and chicken for dinner—relatively cheaply by historical standards—meat production is a different story.

Today, especially for those of us in urban United States and Canada, most of our meat comes from large-scale industrial operations. Often called "factory farms," these mechanized and standardized operations turn out massive quantities of meat. Some people have become dubious about this system, knowing that factory farms crowd animals, afford them limited opportunities for normal behavior, and feed and medicate them for maximum weight gain. We're aware that the system is ethically questionable, despite the argument for plenty at so little cost.

But there is rising evidence of other implications that are more difficult to ignore. Industrial meat production of the type and intensity of today appears to be ecologically impossible long term. It uses a volume of resources and causes a volume of waste that seems beyond the ability of the planet to cope, contributing to a network of environmental and public health problems.

On the input side, factory farming uses staggering amounts of land, fuel, water, fertilizers, and chemicals to grow corn, soy, and other feed crops. On the output side, animal agriculture creates copious greenhouse gases and mountains of manure, some of which ends up contaminating water and soil. Large-scale animal production accelerates climate change, undermines biodiversity, and adds to disease and antibiotic resistance. A resource-intensive food, meat uses large portions of the Earth's arable land and is a factor in the decline of locally controlled family farming worldwide.[1]

Frequently supported and sometimes even subsidized by our governments, industrialized meat production puts bacon, ribs and chicken in grocery stores at prices that encourage us to eat more than is good for us or the planet. But eventually—practically invisibly—we pay the full cost through contaminated water, bacterial infections, animal-to-human flus, and increased rates of obesity, heart disease, strokes, diabetes, and cancers.[2]

I am not suggesting that meat deserves all the blame for our environmental or public health problems. Water pollution, of course, comes from many sources. Industry, domestic waste, and the overuse of pharmaceuticals and pesticides are just a few examples. Greenhouse gases come from air transportation, from construction, from an expanding human population and urbanization, from our over-reliance on cars, and from fuel-dependent international trade. Health problems are the result of myriad interlocking factors, including genes, industrial toxins, cigarettes, and junk food.

But meat production and consumption add markedly to our troubles. Academic and professional researchers, international health agencies, and environmental groups have documented the pressing implications of over-production and over-consumption of animal-source foods, what one book termed "The Meat Crisis."[3]

The problems seem overwhelming, but they're amenable to solutions that every one of us can help bring about. We can feed a growing population while minimizing adverse environmental effects. We can make food that is healthy using production methods that are ecologically tenable for the long term and show regard for animals. Joyce D'Silva, a prominent British researcher who has been writing on meat and livestock issues for decades, says the evidence is clear that we can feed the world in 2050 humanely and sustainably "if we reduce meat consumption."[4]

Addressing Livestock and Meat Is Key to Food Security

Food security has become a concept for our time. A unifying idea in the growing citizen "food movement," food security is a kind of hope. It's an objective, a plan, and even a prayer that humans might figure

out how to provide predictable and widespread access to basic sustenance that is adequate, healthy, and appropriate. The food movement
calls for deep changes in agriculture, including local control over food
systems through "food sovereignty" and "food democracy." The movement is a collage of people and organizations seeking to address major
challenges: global starvation and undernutrition; an epidemic of diet-
related disease; a proliferation of over-processed snacks and meals with
too much salt, fats, and sweeteners; environmental degradation from
chemical-dependent agriculture; and control of food production by
large corporations. The movement for food security argues that current
systems of sustenance aren't serving most of us very well, even those of
us who get served several times a day.

Food security is a compelling area of study and action because it
draws on the biggest challenges of our day. Food is an environmental
issue, a health issue, an ethical issue, and a social justice issue. For all
these reasons, the food movement calls to me, as it calls to many of
you. When I tell people the topic of my research, almost everyone has
a food story or is eager to talk about what's healthy, what's sustainable,
and what they should eat. I am not trained in clinical nutrition and
do not give dietary advice. But I'm drawn to issues that are relevant to
how we eat. I gradually became aware of such issues through my travels
in developing countries[5] and through my research on a wide range of
topics related to my writing and teaching. For ten years, I worked as a
journalist, then studied psychology and neuroscience before spending
another decade as a college instructor teaching about health and illness
of body and mind. Food issues continued to intrigue me, so I signed
on for an additional graduate degree in food policy, which allowed me
to read and learn about what researchers are saying is right and wrong
with the ways we farm and eat today.

My decision to focus on "the meat problem" developed when I realized that, in political and community discussions about food systems,
the topic of animal products didn't seem to get the attention warranted
by the scientific research. You could say that, in public discourse, meat
is rare. Within governments, focus on the problem is almost nonexis-
tent — except when elected officials are required to address short-term

crises such as bacterial infections or animal flus. The topic of meat is seen as "politically explosive," in the words of international food policy expert Dr. Tim Lang who, along with his colleagues, says the meat problem and potential solutions are terrain "which few if any politicians dare to enter."[6] The Food and Agriculture Organization (FAO) of the United Nations calls livestock one of the most crucial, yet least understood, topics of our time that "should rank as one of the leading focuses for environmental policy."[7]

Yet potential solutions to the meat problem aren't radical. There's no need for whole populations to become vegetarian, or for people to stop raising livestock. As you'll see throughout this book, what's needed is a moderate but widespread response by entire households, communities, and nations to decrease consumption of animal products and support producers who are raising livestock within the capacity of local ecosystems. Some people have chosen not to eat meat or other animal-source foods, or will make that choice. But those who wish to include animal products in their diets can do so in moderation and still know they're contributing to health and sustainability.

When I began researching this book five years ago, it was unusual to suggest that people eat less meat. But the movement is growing quickly, and more people have come to agree that we've got a problem and that everyone — vegetarians and meat-eaters alike — can be part of the solution.

Nevertheless, the suggestion that people moderate their consumption has its critics. It's not surprising that much of the criticism for the "eat less meat" message comes from agribusiness, the large corporations that dominate agriculture and food. However, there are also critics from the other side of the table. Some are animal activists who don't believe it's right for humans to consume meat at all. Other critics say that for health reasons we should all just give up animal-source foods.[8] While I sympathize with the concern for the way billions of food animals are treated, I believe that livestock can be raised sustainably and compassionately. I also believe animal-source foods can be healthy in small amounts. Besides, most people aren't willing to make a total break.

I've come across ambivalence, and even antipathy, to this issue from some scientists and activists. Three years ago, I was scolded in front of a large audience by a climate-change scientist who claimed that meat and its environmental consequences constitute a trivial issue promoted by (in his words) ideological vegetarians. A few minutes later, he told me privately he is aware that large-scale meat production is a problem for ecosystems, but will not say so publicly for fear of appearing "marginal."[9] The meat issue is, indeed, a tough sell, and I don't focus on it for my personal comfort. Once you start recommending that people ease back on their meat consumption, some people won't ask you to dinner.[10]

Yet more and more individuals and organizations are agreeing on the importance of the topic. There is a surging chorus of voices calling for animal agriculture that is consistent with our deepest desires to promote the health of our planet and our fellow beings. While conducting this research, I've had the pleasure to connect with policymakers and organizations involved in educating citizens about the need to consume "less and better." These groups promote the idea of producing fewer livestock animals in ways that are more harmonious with the environment and with health in the broadest sense. I've also had the honor to meet and interview Americans and Canadians who work courageously for cleaner and kinder food systems — people you'll encounter as you read this book.

You'll hear about a family in upstate New York that produces sheep, cattle, pigs, and chickens with no hormones or antibiotics. Their animals are raised in numbers low enough to enrich rather than degrade the land. You'll read about an organic beef farmer who believes he has a duty to steward the precious southern Alberta ranchland. There's a southern Ontario woman who runs a mixed organic crop-and-livestock operation who also travels the world speaking in support of sustainable farmers. There's a California chef who shows omnivores how delicious meatless meals can be. There are university-based researchers across the United States, Canada, Europe, and Australia working for more ecological food policies. There are experts at the United Nations FAO, based in Rome, who ignited the debate on the meat problem with a groundbreaking report in 2006. There are scientists in North Carolina and Manitoba who raise awareness of the environmental and health problems of intensive animal factories. There are activists toiling for clean water and air, working hard to educate people about the ecological and ethical questions of intensive livestock. I met ordinary citizens whose quality of life was compromised when a factory farm moved into their neighborhood. Their experiences illustrate the depth and breadth of the meat problem, and the dedication of those who are challenging it.

In Chapter 5, you'll read about plain-speaking Don Webb, a 70-something North Carolinan who was an intensive hog farmer until he realized his animal factory was causing such terrible odors that his rural neighbors couldn't enjoy the outdoors. It made him sell off his hogs and start down a different path, opposing corporations in their quest to expand facilities in his part of the world. Mr. Webb still enjoys his meat, however, and said he was once approached by a supporter of agribusiness. Looking for a chance to embarrass Mr. Webb, the man boomed: "Don, I hear tell you like to eat pork!" Replied Mr. Webb: "Hell, yeah, I love pork. I love ribs and bacon and chitlins." However, he said, he also loves sex, but that doesn't mean he wants a red-light district next door.[11]

I also sought alternative opinions, in particular, from representatives of intensive meat production. Though we may disagree on particular topics, I respect such individuals who are genuine in their desire to provide good food, consistent with government priorities and consumer habits. That said, I and many others believe those government priorities and consumer habits need to be reconsidered.

As individuals and as societies, there are modest and common-sense responses we can make to the seemingly overwhelming food-related issues of access, equity, ecology, and health. As consumers, we can act immediately — at the grocery store, in our kitchens, in restaurants, and in our daily lives. We can commit to eating more meatless meals and smaller portions of animal products. We can choose meat, dairy products, and seafood that have been produced well, and we can be willing to pay more for it. Equally crucial, there are steps our governments can take to strengthen environmental and health guidelines on production, support medium- and small-scale operations, and promote good consumption. These questions are global ones, and ultimately they will need to be addressed multilaterally as well as locally. The changes won't come easily, yet the scale of the meat problem calls for action.

Dairy and fish consumption are also part of the problem, since both are increasing beyond the planet's capacity to cope. I discuss the topic briefly, but concentrate on meat. And, while I do discuss the international situation in this book, I focus on the United States and Canada as key examples of the problem and of potential solutions.

We're Capable of Eating Less and Better

It's easy to be skeptical about people's ability to reduce their meat consumption. I've heard experts give detailed summaries of the devastation to the environment and public health from too many livestock and too much meat, yet some of those same experts continue to assume that heavily meat-centered diets are inevitable. But there are reasons to be optimistic that we can make relatively small adjustments in our lives and large adjustments in our food systems.

People can change, as I learned over the years studying and teaching psychology. We, as individuals, can alter our behavior and habits when they cause us trouble, whether in love or money, work or play. History demonstrates that whole societies can change. Less than 200 years ago, slavery and serfdom were widely accepted practices. And it was only about a century ago that women got the right to vote. And, in a less dramatic example, remember that just a few decades ago, people smoked cigarettes anywhere and anytime — including at the adjoining table in your neighborhood restaurant. There are countless examples of the power of new attitudes. Social norms can change. People can change.

Eating less and better meat is a natural extension of shifts that many of us are already making. More and more people are committing to healthier eating and choosing local and organic foods that are good for the environment and their communities, and there is a small but growing movement among food-conscious people to decrease their intake of animal products. This is laying the groundwork for addressing the meat problem.

Eating less and better meat is consistent with basic values we all hold, whether philosophical, religious, or common sense. We want to act in ways that are good for our families, friends, and communities, and for the people and animals with whom we share the planet. Years ago, we may have thought this could be accomplished by eating as much meat as possible. Today, the evidence suggests a different course.

People who are intrigued about eating less meat increasingly have access to specific strategies, many of which are discussed in this book. The strategies aren't complicated, but are nevertheless important: moving flesh foods to the side of the plate, serving smaller portions, using culinary alternatives, and resolving to buy organic and locally produced chicken, pork, and beef. The meat problem can be addressed top-down by policymakers, but also bottom-up by all of us, as citizens of the world.

I believe these changes are possible. I believe this despite being aware there are powerful forces opposed to changes in food systems and consumer habits. These include agribusinesses that work to convince us we need processed foods and animal products every day. But they also include our evolutionary attraction to high-fat foods, and our comfortable, long-standing dietary habits. Altering these structures and habits will take commitment.

My belief that we can address these problems stems partly from my experience in altering my own food habits. As a teenager, I overate sweets and fast foods, and in adulthood I retained a taste for dishes smothered in heavy sauces. I still occasionally reach for too many chocolate desserts or salt-and-vinegar potato chips. Mostly, however, my eating is moderate and nourishing. I consume small amounts of animal products, including cheese and (very occasionally) a little wild fish. My meals are based on fresh vegetables, grains, legumes, and fruits, plus a small amount of animal products — minimally processed and organic, when possible. I have grown to love brown rice and sautéed vegetables with light sauces allowing the flavor of the food to come through. I occasionally allow myself "fun foods," such as popcorn and beer.

It doesn't matter to me whether someone is "vegetarian," a term people apply to themselves for many different reasons. Sometimes it's because they eat few or no animal products. Sometimes it's because they only eat meat a couple of times a week, or only white meat, or eggs but no dairy, or fish but no chicken. And sometimes they eat all kinds of meat — but feel guilty about it. The proliferation of these flexible definitions gives me confidence that more and more people consider it desirable to be discerning about their intake of animal foods.

Food became a serious concern for me years ago when I read a book describing intensive livestock operations.[12] It jarred me into cutting out meat and starting to view meals in light of the health and well-being of people, of animals, and of the world. Since then, I've gradually developed new eating patterns and discovered that culinary tastes and habits are not immutable.

The fact that I don't eat meat gives me a point of view on issues of livestock. One friend cautioned me to keep it quiet for fear of being accused of bias. Indeed, in one academic article on the health benefits of reduced meat consumption, the author, despite being internationally renowned in the fields of food and health, felt the need to add a footnote that he has no conflict of interest and "is not a vegetarian."[13] We all have points of view and limitations. Me too, including that I'm a city person without intimate personal experience of food production. However, my suggestion that people eat less meat is strongly supported by scientific evidence. As well, I'm not recommending that anyone — let alone, everyone — desist from eating meat. If everyone stopped, it would cause another set of environmental problems, since sustainable agriculture frequently relies on integrating livestock into crop production.

But why would meat-eaters be considered more objective on this topic than non-meat-eaters? Behind much of research, there are points of view. What is important is that our conclusions be based on reliable evidence and the work of recognized experts in the field. Besides, whether I'm a vegetarian or not depends on how you define it. In my opinion, what matters is not labels, but that we all work together for sustainable food systems. Nevertheless, I urge you to form your own opinions and to accept or reject mine guided by your own assessment of the evidence.

Whatever positions we take, I believe and hope we can cooperate to improve food systems. That belief stems from a worldview that life is purposeful and that we need to act as if positive change is possible. From personal experience and from social science research, I have found that people who believe they can make a difference tend to act in ways that cause them to make a difference. So it makes sense to be confident in our ability to help improve the world.

Our confidence, our attitudes and our choices have weighty consequences. I've been haunted by a phrase from Herman Melville, who said that to produce a mighty book you must have a mighty theme. This book does not aspire to be mighty, but its theme qualifies. Today's large-scale production of livestock, and the storm of problems it brings, is one of the great challenges and decision points of our time. Let's call this a meaty book with a meaty theme. And, if you'll allow me one more pun (discussions of meat are full of them), the book is also about stakes. It's about flesh steaks, but it's also about the high stakes for the planet and humanity. It's about lowering the steaks.

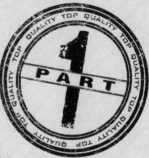

WHY?

REASONS FOR EATING LESS MEAT

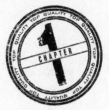

WE'RE ON A BINGE

"...Now I eat meat twice a day."

Whether we live in the city or the countryside, most of us couldn't possibly guess how many livestock animals live on planet Earth. That's because today, it's possible to stand in the middle of livestock country and not see a cow, or a chicken, or a pig. I got an aerial view of this odd absence when I flew in a light plane over pig country in both North Carolina and Manitoba. The land is agricultural, with green and brown acreages stretching to the horizon, yet actual animals are difficult to spot. What you can see are row upon row of long, windowless buildings, each housing thousands of animals big enough to be labeled "hogs." Here, as in much of the industrialized world today, livestock animals are largely invisible. But the poultry and cattle and pigs are with us nonetheless, and not by the thousands, but by the millions, billions, and tens of billions.

Livestock now far outnumber humans on the globe. At any one moment, the number of meat and milk animals is roughly 25 billion, according to the United Nations' Food and Agriculture Organization (FAO).[1] Compare that with seven billion people, and you'll find that there are more than three livestock animals for every one of us. Here's an even more dramatic number to consider: in any given year, more than

50 billion animals are killed for food.[2] There are so many beasts among us that some scientists have coined the phrase "the livestock revolution" to describe the growing centrality of animal foods to human life.[3]

There are tens of billions of livestock animals around the world because we're on a meat binge. We're on a production binge, cranking out hundreds of millions of tons of chicken, beef, and pork each year.[4] And we're on a consumption binge. More of us, more often, are carving into a substantial piece of flesh at the center of our mealtime plates. Never before have humans made meat so integral to their diets and their lives. Not simply the reflection of a growing human population, much of the rise in meat consumption is per capita. On average, each person on the planet is eating more meat than did most of our ancestors.

You may be surprised to hear that global meat production and consumption are on the increase. Your meat-centered meals may seem similar to those of your parents and grandparents, and for your family that may be true, since in wealthy countries some of the leap in meat consumption occurred several generations ago. As well, you probably know a few vegetarians and perhaps some individuals who say they have moderated their meat intake for health, ethical, or environmental reasons. There is, indeed, a small but growing trend for less red meat and even less meat overall.[5] Per capita meat consumption has been declining slightly in the United States for a few years now.[6] But for most people, flesh foods continue to be the star of the meal. Even when consumers say they want to eat better for the environment and their health, they cut down on beef, but often eat chicken as a substitute.[7] Americans consume, on average, three to four times as much meat per capita as the typical African citizen, and roughly twice the overall global amount.[8] The average American tucks away enough meat in a year to equal the weight of a large person — around 200 pounds.[9] Consumers may be starting to rethink the binge, but an observation from the US Department of Agriculture a decade ago still holds: "Now more than ever, America is a nation of meat-eaters."[10]

Citizens of other industrialized nations aren't far behind. On average, consumers in developed nations take in the daily equivalent of two large burgers, 200 to 250 grams (about 7–9 ounces) or more, some in actual ground round, but most in chicken, pork, and other beef cuts.[11] For many families, in many parts of the world, it is considered normal to have pork, chicken, or beef every day and sometimes at every meal. In addition, seafood and dairy products have become dramatically larger additions to our diets.

Year-over-year increases in meat consumption are particularly striking in developing and emerging economies. But for decades all over the world, people have been deriving more and more calories from animal products, and international meat production is predicted to more than double between 2000 and 2050.[12] As one middle-aged Asian man remarked to me in conversation: "When I was a child, we ate meat twice a week. Now I eat it twice a day."

We're Climbing the Food Chain to Dangerous Heights

Meat has long been part of the human diet.[13] Hunting and meat-eating have influenced human history, requiring cooperative behavior and giving people sources of dense nutrients. Some scientists suggest that meat consumption encouraged human brain development, in part because even partial flesh-food diets require less intestinal tract action and metabolic energy than purely herbivorous diets, freeing more energy for cognition. But whatever positive role meat may have played historically, and however useful meat may be, it has not always made a large contribution to overall sustenance. Humans are omnivores capable of surviving on a wide range of diets, including vegetarian ones, and animal-source foods have often played roles of mere dietary condiment or occasional luxury.

There have been times and places in which humans had meaty diets. Think of far-northern peoples who survived largely on seal and other animal flesh. Our hunter-gatherer ancestors may have received one third or more of their sustenance from animal products.[14] But in times past, the meat was wild or traditionally grown, was leaner and more natural than today, contained no antibiotics or chemicals, and was complemented by high-fiber plant matter, not processed foods.

With the Industrial Revolution of the 18th and 19th centuries, traditional methods of doing just about everything were reexamined as candidates for mass production. Soon, people had access to industrially made foods. Over the past 250 years in England, the per capita consumption of fat and sugar has soared. Between the 18th and 19th centuries in Europe, per-person consumption of meat multiplied 100 times.[15] That's not 100% more; it's 100 times more.

The trend continued during the second half of the 20th century, when mass production was increasingly applied to livestock. World meat production increased fourfold between 1961 and 2006.[16] Part of that increase was simply to accommodate a growing human population, but part was due to the fact that the average person on the planet increased their meat intake during that half century.

This massive dietary change has been occurring for decades. Often called the "nutrition transition,"[17] the shift sounds benign but describes the tendency for billions of people to choose fewer homegrown and traditional meals, more processed foods, sugars, fats, and salt, and considerably more meat, dairy products, and fish. The transition has brought variety and nutrients to the poorest of the world. But it has also seen whole populations move away from natural, locally sourced foods toward factory-made ones, and away from plant-based diets toward diets heavy on animal foods. The nutrition transition is also intertwined with rising material standards of living, since livestock also provide byproducts such as fats and gelatins for consumer products, natural animal hormones for human drugs, and animal skin for leathers.[18]

Dairy is part of the dietary stampede up the food chain. In many parts of the world, people are consuming increasing amounts of milk, cheese, yogurt, and ice cream. Over the past few decades, milk intake has been climbing steadily, especially in developing countries — and that's per capita.[19] Let's emphasize the term "per capita," which is not just a statistical concept but means that, on average, every single citizen of the world (particularly in poor countries) is consuming much more milk than residents did a generation ago.

Incredibly, the world over, there is now twice as much milk consumed (by weight) each year as all meat products.[20] Milk is the source of more and more calories, even in parts of the world where people have not traditionally eaten much dairy. India, China, and other countries

are developing a taste for Western-style butter and cheese, supporting
the projection that worldwide milk production will double between the
years 2000 and 2050.[21]

Fish also illustrate the lure of animal products to a degree impossible to maintain in the long term.[22] Aquatic animals now form such a
large part of the human diet that global stocks are in crisis. Experts not
given to hyperbole regularly refer to an impending collapse of fish species. The United Nations reports that one third of fish supplies are over-
exploited or depleted. For large sea animals such as tuna, as many as
90% have been depleted in the past half century, and more than half of
tuna species are at risk of extinction.[23] Atlantic cod have been harvested
to near disappearance, as has bluefin tuna. The Newfoundland cod fish-
ery has declined dramatically from pressures including industrial-scale
fishing.[24] A friend likes to joke that he didn't arrive at the top of the
food chain in order to eat tofu. But are billions of humans climbing the
food chain too high?

There's a Push for Mass Production and Consumption

Why the massive changes in our eating habits? Why do we expect animal products at almost every meal? In part, simply because it is there,
and at prices most people can afford. Meat is widely available today — at
the grocery store, the corner restaurant, and every fast-food chain —
at relative prices below what previous generations paid. During some
holiday seasons, my local supermarket has turkey for 99 cents a pound,
and this week, a nearby fast-food outlet is selling burgers for $1.50.
Today, Americans spend 2% of their annual income to buy 221 pounds
of red meat and poultry, whereas 40 years ago they spent 4% of their
income to obtain only 194 pounds.[25]

Loads of meat at low prices is a result of the rise and industry dominance of factory farms. Officially called "confined (or concentrated) animal feeding operations" (CAFOs), or "intensive livestock operations"
(ILOs), they're more factory than farm, and they are the source of most
of the meat available to most people in the United States and Canada.
CAFOs and ILOs, applying the principles of mass manufacturing to
livestock, raise thousands of animals indoors using mechanization and

technology for maximum production. CAFOs are defined by US officials as operations that confine at least 1,000 beef cattle, or 700 dairy cows, or 2,500 large swine, or 125,000 broiler chickens.[26] CAFO systems fatten the animals quickly then later send them down mechanized disassembly lines to be chopped and wrapped in cellophane.

Factory farm operators care about the animals, and care for them as best they can. But it's difficult to give them healthy and humane care when you're trying to produce as much meat as quickly as possible — and when the chickens and pigs are packed tight in buildings or cages in a system that philosopher and animal-welfare expert Bernard Rollin calls "the end of animal husbandry."[7] Virginia-based farmer Joel Salatin is a vocal critic of many of the ways we live today, including our reliance on industrial meat, egg, and dairy production. To make his point, Mr. Salatin entitled his latest book *Folks, This Ain't Normal*.[28] He's right that current systems are not normal by historical standards. Our ancestors ate the meat of animals that had been raised on pasture, grass, or scraps from farmyards and family kitchens. In contrast, much of our meat today comes from factory farms. Worldwide, ILOs or CAFOs produce at least 75% of all poultry, 40% of all pork, more than two thirds of all eggs, and a significant amount of the beef we consume.[29] Those percentages are higher in the United States, Canada, Europe, and other wealthy regions. Food systems writer David Kirby says that for us "the vast majority of pigs, chickens, and dairy cows are produced inside animal factories."[30] And, as we'll see in Chapter 5, the concentration of animals indoors has been paralleled by the concentration of meat-sector ownership in the hands of just a few corporations.

Before reading widely on these topics, I had assumed that factory farms, despite their environmental problems, were more economically efficient than small livestock producers. Yet, analyses of the meat sector suggest that cost-effectiveness is not the main reason intensive industrial production dominates the world of meat and milk. In addition to employing advances in technology, CAFOs have the advantages of scale, so they benefit from the economic principle of spreading costs over larger numbers of widgets — in this case servings of meat. But factory farms, and the agribusinesses that own them, have the additional

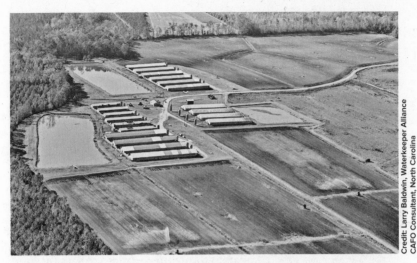

Credit: Larry Baldwin, Waterkeeper Alliance
CAFO Consultant, North Carolina

Confined Animal Feeding Operations (CAFOs), or factory farms, in eastern North Carolina. Each building can house thousands of animals. On the left side of the photo are two "lagoons" or outdoor storage pits for manure and urine. Near the bottom of the photo are machines spraying the waste onto fields.

advantage of support from our governments. "When examined in detail, economies of scale largely disappear for CAFOs," says researcher Doug Gurian-Sherman of the Union of Concerned Scientists. "A more important factor is processor-driven vertical integration and coordination, and the resulting accumulation of market power in the hands of large processors."[31]

The trend to industrialization and concentration has developed over years of direct and indirect support for technological ways of doing things.[32] First, a series of farm bills lowered the prices of crops used as feed for intensive livestock. Second, environmental authorities declined to strongly enforce pollution control from factory farms. Third, federal justice officials allowed numerous corporate mergers. Such policies have shaped the sector to be what it is today, and have allowed for artificially low retail prices that encourage heavy consumption and fail to account for livestock's ultimate costs to the environment and our health.[33] Meanwhile, size alone does not determine efficiency in livestock production, and studies show that well-managed small and medium-sized operations can be as cost-efficient as some CAFOs.[34] That's especially true when you factor in the manure that CAFOs impose on ecosystems, and the resulting health and environmental damage. When all costs and benefits are tallied, small and medium livestock operations are probably preferable economically as well as environmentally.

But agribusiness is influential, as illustrated by the very benefits it receives from favorable legislation. Factory farms are generally not required to adhere to strict animal-welfare standards, and they are often protected by exemptions allowing practices that are common in agriculture today.[35] A number of states are moving to limit the ability of citizens to photograph factory farms.[36] Some jurisdictions have food libel laws, also called "agricultural products disparagement laws," which make it easier for food companies to sue their critics.[37] That's the kind of legislation that put TV personality Oprah Winfrey in court in the late 1990s after a televised conversation about beef in the wake of the mad cow scare. Ms. Winfrey eventually won her case, but not until the public got a lesson in the power of industrial food.

Excessive Supply Drives Excessive Demand

Most people like the taste of meat and enjoy hotdogs and chicken wings, but those precise preferences aren't genetic or otherwise inevitable. We come into the world craving foods high in calories, but not necessarily animal foods. Over time, we learn to choose specific ways to satisfy our cravings, influenced by practical considerations such as what is available and the social messages we receive. We're not always consciously aware of the messages, but have years of memories from home, television, and media ads of people declaring how delicious the meat is. We also gravitate toward animal products as signs of worldliness and success. When hosting for guests, most of us would not consider serving a meal in which meat was not the main attraction, even if we were aware of excellent plant-based cuisine. Whether or not people have heard of the Italian *cucina povera* ("food of the poor"), they tend to feel that cabbage and potatoes are less worthy than veal and prime rib.[38]

Yet such perceptions can be amplified by marketing, and here is where demand meets supply. The livestock revolution is often labeled primarily "demand-driven,"[39] implying that consumers have clamored for more, forcing producers to make more. Natural demand does indeed play a role. But just as big consumption needs big production, so high-volume industrial production needs enthusiastic buyers. Once intensive livestock systems started churning it out, agribusiness needed customers to believe that meat was a daily essential. The meat binge is not just demand-driven, it is also supply-driven.

Intensive ad campaigns for both brand-name and generic meats and products are potent in their ability to increase consumer demand.[40] Galloping meat intake, according to top international climate-change scientist Dr. Rajendra Pachauri, is a result partly of increased incomes but also of "very effective marketing strategies pursued by the industry."[41] Meat can also be promoted through other channels such as government dietary guidelines and advice, which in turn can be influenced by industry, as will be shown in Chapter 9. As documented by nutrition professor and renowned food systems analyst Marion Nestle, meat agribusiness employs lobbyists to keep consumers and policymakers thinking positively and to "make sure that no government agency ever says, 'Eat less meat.'"[42]

Massive and concentrated production was never supposed to create problems; it was supposed to solve them. From the early to the mid-20th century, policy experts around the world searched for ways to feed populations reliably and to avoid crises such as the widespread hunger of the 1930s[43] (vividly evoked in John Steinbeck's *The Grapes of Wrath*[44]) and the periodic famines that have occurred throughout human history. Experts understandably believed that what was needed was volume. So nations began shaping food systems for large productive capacity. By the mid-20th century, after two world wars and the Depression, satisfying people's basic needs was top priority. Industrial systems seemed a good idea, and the more food factories the better. Few people at that time would have imagined the possibility that there could be too much of any food.

Yet today, as the prototype of industrial food, modern meat systems have contributed to problems previously unforeseen. They have helped persuade billions of consumers to strive for a constant stream of animal-source foods. In today's volumes, raising livestock exhausts the planet, overuses land and fresh water, and adds to climate change. Modern meat pollutes water and is a factor in avian flus and other serious problems, as I'll describe in later chapters. Once meat is made, the amount of it we eat can also undermine human health.

It's not the cattle or the hogs that are the problem, but the number of them that now exist. The problem is not that we eat chicken, pork, or beef, but that we consume so much of it. Making and eating small amounts can be good for the planet and human well-being, but today it's a different story. A question of scale, meat is also on a weigh scale being balanced against environment, health, and community.

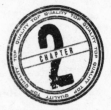

Too Many Livestock Compromise Land and Climate

Meat Should Make Environmental Sense

In theory, keeping livestock is an ecologically sensible idea. Animals can roam over rough acreage that is neither particularly arable for crops nor good for human settlement, or they can live among small-scale farms and human communities. If they're cattle, sheep, or goats, they survive nicely on tough grasses that are inedible to people, and if they're pigs or chickens, they can root and peck for wild plants and scraps. They leave manure as fertilizer and provide milk, meat, and leather, supplying services and materials humans need — from virtually nothing. Livestock were raised this way traditionally, and they still are here and there, of necessity in remote regions and deliberately in organic and low-density operations. For some peoples, animals are part of the natural world and their centuries-old practice of living in balance with that world. But however sensible such practices are, they can't produce billions of cut-rate and standardized servings each year, especially for urbanites living far from the source. As a result, in the United States, Canada, and around the world, production is now dominated by large-scale intensive production facilities — among the most environmentally costly ways to make food.

The costs begin with that most tangible of resources: land. Agriculture has always affected the land, as humans drained swamps and chopped down forests to plant crops. When in past generations we damaged land irrevocably, we could generally expand our way out of the problem.[1] We could find new land on the frontier. But with seven billion of us and growing, and with much of global land occupied and little left in the way of frontier, this time we may be in a bind. Where land is concerned, as a realtor friend of mine likes to say, "they're not making any more of it." As a result, the way we produce meat may be difficult or impossible to maintain for the long term — the very definition of unsustainable. Central to that is large-scale meat production's voracious appetite for land.

Intensive livestock facilities don't appear to use much land, with animals wing-to-wing or shoulder-to-shoulder in compact buildings. But those billions of animals need to be fed, and the soy, wheat, corn, and barley they eat needs to be grown somewhere. As a result, large portions of the planet are now devoted to growing not food but feed, and it's not for people but for animals. Of all arable terrain on the planet, a full one third is used to grow feed crops.[2] Combine that amount with all the acreages for pasture, and you find that livestock directly or indirectly use 70% of agricultural land and 30% of the entire solid surface of the globe.[3]

Of the large chunk of planetary land now devoted to livestock, much of it used to be either forest or small acreages operated by local farmers to sustain themselves, their families, and their neighbors — organically, of course, the only way anyone farmed before industrial agriculture. Today, forests are disappearing, and land is being overtaken, in part to satisfy our appetite for daily meat.

We've all driven through rural areas and enjoyed the sight of the breeze through the grain and corn, and imagined those crops as sturdy breads on family tables. But we don't see their other destinations. Worldwide, up to three quarters of soybeans, half the corn, and one third of all grains go not to people, but to livestock.[4] That's without even counting the fish that become feed. Most people would be alarmed to know that more than a third of the world fisheries' catch is ground up into fishmeal and oil that is used mostly to fatten pigs, chickens, and farmed fish.[5] This, despite the fact that marine stocks are declining dramatically and some ocean species are near collapse.

Of all the feed swallowed by livestock, much of it doesn't even turn directly into meat or milk, but simply keeps the animals standing, breathing, and chewing. So one ton of feed does not create one ton of meat, but considerably less. If the animals were eating scraps, waste food, or wild grasses, it wouldn't be inefficient. But modern meat production maintains animals on grains and legumes that people themselves could eat, or it is often cultivated on land that could grow food for people.

Making meat — given the amounts and production methods of today — uses far more resources than does making similar quantities of plant foods. Whether brisket or bacon, ribs or wings, milk or cheese, livestock products are resource-intensive. More land is used to make a pound of steak, or even chicken, than to make a pound of vegetables. More energy and fresh water is required to produce meat-based meals than meals on the plant-based end of the spectrum.[6] There are a lot of ways to calculate this, and one study showed that it takes 11 times as much energy to make animal protein as it takes to make the same amount of grain protein.[7] It is reasonable to question whether sacrificing this much land, water, and energy is really a sensible idea.

Livestock Today Casts a Long Shadow

Henning Steinfeld and his colleagues set out to pull together the scientific data on a growing problem — the ecological consequences or footprint of growing animals for food.[8] But when Dr. Steinfeld and his crew published *Livestock's Long Shadow: Environmental Issues and Options,*[9] it had an impact way beyond science, and beyond what they would have imagined. In November 2006, when I and others around the world saw inbox messages announcing the report, then read it, we were stunned. Never before had a document so thoroughly assessed the role of meat and dairy production in global warming and other daunting ecological challenges of our time.

I had a chance to visit Dr. Steinfeld not long after the release of the report. Chief of the Livestock Information, Sector Analysis and Policy Branch of the United Nations Food and Agricultural Organization (FAO) in Rome, he has the unassuming office and manner of a serious agricultural economist. Yet he and the report have become central to a storm of discussion about meat. The publication has been cited by everyone from international authorities to neighborhood vegan activists — some of whom have relied on it to argue that everyone should stop eating animal-source foods. This was not the intention of the authors, whose main argument is for better policy.[10]

Livestock's Long Shadow — 400 pages and weighty in both size and expertise — is not bedtime reading. Full of charts and graphs, it takes motivation to get through it. But even if you read just the Executive Summary, you'll see why it caused a stir. Raising livestock in the numbers we do today, says the report, has overrun the globe, caused land degradation and desertification, polluted soil and air, drained and contaminated water systems, undermined plant and animal biodiversity, and exacerbated illness and disease.[11] "The livestock sector," it concludes, "emerges as one of the top two or three most significant contributors to the most serious environmental problems, at every scale from local to global."[12]

But what may be the report's most alarming revelations concern the connection between meat and climate change. Livestock around the world are responsible for 18% — almost one fifth — of human-caused greenhouse gases (GHGs), and so are serious contributors to global warming.[13] At the scale of production today, livestock are a major factor in a defining environmental crisis of our time.

Livestock's Long Shadow was arresting for what it said and who said it. Not only is the FAO the global center for expertise on food, it is a mainstream body not generally out looking for trouble. The FAO answers to the World Bank and powerful national governments. Yet its report criticized the networks designed and promoted by these bodies, and declared that, worldwide, systems for the production of meat and milk are untenable in the long run for the environment and public health.

There's been plenty of criticism from the meat sector of the FAO report, which agribusiness representatives like to say has been disproven.[14] But many subsequent researchers have strongly supported the FAO's basic evidence and the analysis that led to the conclusion that livestock take a large environmental toll. As one later academic report argued, making meat adds so much to global warming that the topic deserves our full attention. "For the world's higher-income populations, greenhouse gas emissions from meat-eating warrant the same scrutiny as do those from driving and flying."[15]

Meat industry supporters also claim that the authors of *Livestock's Long Shadow* have retracted their figures.[16] It's true that FAO authors backed off from one statement — that livestock emissions contribute "a higher share than transport" to planetary greenhouse gases,[17] conceding that their conclusion was not based on a rigorous comparison.[18] But to reject the report because of one questionable statement is like deciding never to read a newspaper again because of an error on an inside page. *Livestock's Long Shadow* was groundbreaking in the best sense, alerting the world to a serious problem that was little understood and amassing powerful evidence for adding meat to the environmental agenda.

Industry's displeasure is to some degree a general one; they contend that this report and others like it have undermined public confidence in the ecology and health of animal agriculture. That's not fair, says industry: well-managed livestock can be good for the environment and human well-being.[19] According to the American Meat Institute, producers are encouraged to conserve resources, prevent pollution, and upgrade technology for better environmental stewardship, and companies are working to improve practices.[20] Beef is lowering its carbon footprint, says the industry, and the United States is a leader in sustainable beef production.[21]

Of course, industry is right that livestock can be good for the environment, and meat can be good for health, and officials at the UN and around the world don't necessarily disagree. Most of the parties involved in this growing global discussion are not anti-livestock or anti-meat. But many insist it is imperative that we raise animals in ways that don't add to ecosystem degradation.

Meanwhile, precisely how much greenhouse gas comes from live-stock depends on where and how you're measuring it. Within individual industrialized nations like the United States, livestock cause consider-ably less than 18% of greenhouse gases, but this percentage is relative to their large amounts of emissions from transportation, manufacturing, and other uses of energy. In some countries, like New Zealand, live-stock account for considerably more than 18% of total emissions. One group of scientists, from the University of California at Davis, wrote a lengthy report arguing that livestock and meat in the United States contribute only a small percentage of human-caused GHGs.[22] In sup-port of this argument, the American meat industry points out that it is working to decrease GHGs and usefully employ waste for purposes such as energy generation. On the other hand, some scientists claim that the FAO underestimated the problem[23] and that mitigation strate-gies aren't being employed quickly enough. The FAO's global figure may be low, especially today, since livestock numbers continue to climb and since in some ways the report used conservative estimates for livestock emissions. Whatever the exact percentage of human-made gas emis-sions from livestock, research converges on the idea that we can't keep making meat using conventional methods and in current amounts.[24] *Livestock's Long Shadow* remains the authority on global environmental problems from animal agriculture, and it's a call to action on the prob-lem of meat.

It's Deforestation and It's Gas Production

When experts say that meat production results in dangerous climate change, they're referring to the global warming of the Earth and atmo-sphere that is melting polar ice, raising sea levels, and increasing the incidence of floods and other extreme weather events. The vast ma-jority of scientists agree on the urgent nature of climate change and its probable human consequences, which include hunger, conflict, and social chaos.[25]

Global warming is an exacerbation of the naturally benign green-house effect. Normally, gases such as water vapor and carbon dioxide (CO_2) trap heat from the sun and provide a stable average surface temperature of about 14 degrees C — just toasty enough to be comfortable for life on Earth. But since the start of the Industrial Revolution, human ingenuity and ambition have accelerated the creation of greenhouse gases, shoved nature out of balance, and pushed up global temperatures. The problem has been summarized in detail by the Intergovernmental Panel on Climate Change (IPCC), whose scientists agree that human choices and behaviors are "very likely" responsible for most of the warming observed over the past 50 years.[26] Human activities, primarily the burning of fossil fuels and clearing of forests, have greatly intensified normal processes, says the IPCC.[27] "Since the start of the industrial era, about 1750, the overall effect of human activities on climate has been a warming one. The human impact on climate greatly exceeds that due to known changes in natural processes, such as solar changes and volcanic eruptions."[28] Human-made greenhouse gases are mostly carbon dioxide, methane, and nitrous oxide, and it turns out that a hearty portion of these come from agriculture, and most of that comes from livestock.[29]

Meaty contributions to climate change can be summarized in a few short words: deforestation and gas production. When I speak to students on this topic, I often repeat those words to encapsulate the mountain of data and information that's out there. Deforestation and gas production. There is overlap between the two, as you'll see, but I'll discuss them one by one.

Deforestation is just one of the tragic environmental events that most of us don't associate with steak. But the pressure for feed puts pressure on forests, which get cut and burned to make room for pasture and feed crops. Livestock is now the main ingredient in the destruction of tropical rainforest in the fragile Amazon. The international environmental organization Greenpeace has shown that cattle are responsible for 80% of Amazon deforestation.[30] Every few seconds, an entire acre of that forest is lost to cattle ranchers. The FAO concurs and unequivocally calls the livestock industry "the major driver of deforestation."[31] Of the huge swaths of flattened Amazonian rainforest, most is now cattle pasture, and much of the rest is devoted to feed crops. Soy is the largest crop on arable land in Brazil — and it's not grown for tofu burgers. Globally, more than 97% of all soymeal is fed to livestock, mostly chickens and pigs.[32] And soymeal is the largest product of cultivated soybeans, which are partly oil, but about three quarters meal.[33]

Deforestation is environmentally stressful for a number of reasons. Under natural conditions, trees take in carbon dioxide and store it in their roots, trunks, stems, and leaves. A constant cycling of leaves, branches, and other material through the soil maintains a rich ecosystem of fungi, insects, worms, roots, and microbes that stores a lot of carbon. When forests get burned or cleared, much of that bountiful carbon gets sent into the atmosphere.[34] And what replaces the forest is often cropland, specifically, monocultures — vast acreages of single species — that store nowhere near the amount of carbon that the forest did. There's not much complex biomass in a monoculture.[35] Deforestation also exacerbates climate change in another way: by removing trees that would naturally be taking in carbon dioxide from the atmosphere and replacing it with oxygen. When we have fewer trees, we have less capacity to mitigate climate change.

Deforestation therefore worsens global warming, and it makes the problem even harder to solve. So, what scientists call "land-use changes" (mostly deforestation, but also other types of destruction after the forest is gone) put a lot of carbon dioxide into the air in ways that are attributable to livestock and meat.

The second major contribution to climate change from meat is gas production. Although beans have a reputation as a gassy food, that reputation should really belong to meat. Livestock produce gases beyond those released through deforestation. The complicated meat supply-chain sends CO_2 into the atmosphere from mechanized processes on factory farms as well as fossil fuels used for transport and refrigeration. But livestock is also a major source of two additional greenhouse gases: methane and nitrous oxide, both of which are much more potent than carbon dioxide. Methane (CH_4) has a global warming potential (GWP) of 25–72, meaning that each molecule of methane has that many times greater capacity to alter climate than does one molecule of CO_2.[36] Nitrous oxide (N_2O) has a GWP that is even more damaging, at almost 300 times that of CO_2.[37]

Methane wafts largely from cows, sheep, and goats — ruminants whose digestive processes cause them to belch. (Cow flatulence is also a result, but the more significant amount of methane comes from burps.) When the animals feed on fibrous plants, the plants ferment in ruminants' stomachs and methane is produced as a by-product.[38] Decomposing manure yields yet more methane, especially when the waste is stored in liquid form.[39] It's a common practice at factory farms, especially at industrial pig and dairy operations, to hold waste in lagoons, tanks, or pits that sit open to the atmosphere as a bubbling soup.[40]

Nitrous oxide, the other powerful livestock gas, is also a by-product of livestock manure. In addition, it comes from nitrogen fertilizers applied to feed crops and pastureland.[41] Especially because crops are often saturated with more fertilizer than they need,[42] nitrous oxide levels rise invisibly, but continually, across our rural regions. And since many of the crops cultivated in the central United States are for animal feed,[43] it's easy to see that much of the excess nitrous oxide in the ecosystem is tied to the production of large amounts of animal-source foods.

It's easy to feel intimidated by the science of climate change. But the story of how livestock add to global warming comes down largely to deforestation and gas production. There's carbon dioxide from deforestation for pasture and feed crops, from on-farm use of fossil fuels, from transport, and from refrigeration. There's methane from the burps of cattle, sheep, and goats, and from the plentiful manure of all animals. Then there's nitrous oxide from livestock waste and from crop fertilizers. When it's all added up by the FAO, worldwide, livestock are responsible for 9% of human-made carbon dioxide, 37% of methane, and a full 65% of nitrous oxide.[44] That's a lot of global warming from meat.

You may have noticed that the main culprits scientists have identified for meaty GHGs do not include fossil fuels used to truck the food to your table. That's because the majority of gaseous emissions from agriculture — especially for animal products — occur in the initial production stage, not in transport.[45] In dairy production, at least 78% of emissions, and sometimes more than 90%, occur before the food leaves the farm.[46] One report surprised activists by showing that 83% of food-related greenhouse gas emissions result from making the food in the first place, while its transportation — from farmer to your local grocer to your table — is responsible for only 11% of food-related emissions.[47] So, while eating locally produced food is highly desirable for a range of environmental and social reasons, we need to pay attention not only to how far the food has traveled, but to what kind of food it is. In other words, we need to ask how resource-intensive our meals are, if we want to eat sustainably.

In Large Numbers, All Livestock Add to Climate Change

Beef has a bad reputation. After hearing all the media reports on issues ranging from mad cow disease to saturated fats, people who know that meat production adds to global warming assume beef is to blame. Red meat does result in more gases per pound of food than does chicken or fish. But when there are too many animals to be supported by eco-systems, all livestock add dangerously to greenhouse gases and other environmental problems.

Livestock can be categorized either as ruminants (cattle, sheep, and goats) or as monogastrics (pigs and poultry). Ruminants add to green-house gases in several ways. As discussed above, they release methane during digestion. Environmentally, ruminants have an additional strike against them. They need to consume more food than do other species to produce each pound of meat. One pound of beef or lamb on your dinner plate required 10 pounds or more of feed, while one pound of chicken needed almost 2 pounds of feed, and one pound of pork needed roughly 5 pounds of feed, based on what's called feed conversion ratios.[48] So it takes a fair amount of plant material to make a slab of meat, especially red meat. On the plus side, cows and sheep have the ecological advantage of being able to eat tough grasses that humans can't. However, for much of ruminant production, that's just theory. Although cattle and sheep are happiest on grass, most raised for wealthy countries are fattened, for at least part of their lives, on industrially produced rations, such as grain, corn, or soy. After a few months on pasture, they're sent to feedlots to beef up on concentrated calories. I've seen this in feedlot regions where thousands of cattle stand crowded in pens, dipping their snouts into troughs to get their fill.

Pigs and poultry don't have ruminant digestive systems, so they don't burp methane. But they have their own ways of adding to climate change. They're not designed to eat natural, tough grasses like the ruminants are, and in modern meat production they don't live on food scraps and wild plants. But they've got to eat something. So billions of chickens and pigs are given cereals, soy, corn, and other crops, all of which require land, water, pesticides, and fertilizers that exact a toll on ecosystems.

Dairy products are not as obvious in their climate-change potential. But when one considers the large and growing amount of milk-based food consumed around the world, the challenge to the environment becomes clear. Milk comes from ruminants — animals that breathe out greenhouse gases as well as making manure. Most of the livestock methane on Earth (and a large percentage of all direct greenhouse gases) comes from cattle raised for meat or milk.[49] So, reducing your meat consumption isn't as environmentally effective if you just replace it with large amounts of cheese. Some researchers calculate beef as the most significant livestock contributor to greenhouse gases, with milk in second place, then pigs, then poultry.[50] But per pound of food produced, milk products don't look so bad. Milk can be drawn from animals continually, while meat, of course, is obtained only at an animal's death. As a result, while dairy cows belch and defecate into the environment, meanwhile they provide a lot of food. To lower greenhouse gases, it does help to reduce consumption of dairy products, but it helps more to reduce servings of flesh foods.[51]

When you directly compare species, it's true that red meats add most to climate change. They're responsible for roughly 1.5 times as much GHG per pound of food produced as chicken or fish.[52] According to some researchers, sheep and beef meats have the worst climate impacts, at more than twice that of pigs or poultry.[53] Pound for pound, though, lamb is actually the biggest offender, but since it makes up only about 1% of meat consumed in the United States, its aggregate emissions aren't so bad.[54] Beef, as the prototype red meat making up almost one third of our meat intake, racks up most of the numbers. Yet all animals need to eat, and all of them make manure that emits powerful methane and nitrous oxide gases. One bit of good news is that chickens are the smallest contributors to greenhouse gases per unit of meat produced,[55] and they're the most numerous livestock animal on the planet today. Yet when there are tens of billions, all animals add dangerously to greenhouse gases. Even for beef, the problem isn't the cattle themselves, but the number we produce and the amount we eat. Like other meats, we could eat it sustainably, if we made it carefully and ate it sparingly.

Cows and other ruminants add to climate change even when they're raised naturally on grassy rangeland. In fact, supporters of intensive livestock production point out that grass-fed ruminants can in some cases emit even more methane (per pound of meat produced) than factory-farmed ones.[56] However, that doesn't mean intensively raised beef are better for the planet overall. Feedlots and other CAFOs produce voluminous manure in confined areas, require tons of feed that exacted environmental costs to grow and transport, and administer pharmaceuticals that end up in the environment. The fact that even naturally raised beef cattle emit greenhouse gases is yet another argument for lowering the numbers of ruminants globally, however they're produced.

At the heart of the issue is the reality that producing meat emits more greenhouse gases than producing plant foods. This has been demonstrated in many studies.[57] The latest to come across my desk analyzed the GHGs of 61 categories of foods and beverages, and it showed that meat and dairy products produce far more gases, per pound, than do most other edibles.[58] Cut down on meat and dairy, and you'll be helping cut down on greenhouse gases.

When you do eat less meat, you'll need to consume something else instead. So what are the climate-change costs of producing substitute foods?

Researchers warn that "default" or "substitute" emissions might end up being high,[59] and that we won't just erase 18% of GHGs by cutting back on meat. How much good we do for the environment partly depends on the substitutes we choose. When we simply go for more vegetables, whole grains, legumes, and fruits, we're saving significant GHGs. But many people enjoy meat alternatives like the veggie sausages to which I occasionally treat myself for weekend breakfasts. They're solid and satisfying foods, and some look and taste like animal products, which is appealing to some consumers. Meat substitutes are useful, and are fine in moderation. But those that are highly processed — often precisely to make them look or taste like flesh food — can be environmentally costly.[60] There's nothing wrong with a few treats, but the most ecological meal plate is one piled with minimally processed grains, vegetables, legumes, or fruits — edibles with small "food-prints." The idea that various foods can have an impact on climate change was voiced a decade ago by experts from Johns Hopkins Bloomberg School of Public Health when they said: "One personal act that can have a profound impact on these issues is reducing meat consumption."[61]

Wealthy Countries Need to Lower Consumption

Factory farms may produce most of the meat in industrialized countries, but they're not the only livestock problem on the planet. All over the world, animals are being raised in ways that deplete land and resources and worsen climate change. This includes "extensive" livestock production based on grazing, as well as "intensive" factory production.

Speaking broadly, there are three ways to raise livestock: grazing or grassland-based (extensive), mixed crop-and-livestock, and factory farming (intensive).[62] The first two systems are the most natural ones and have long existed in human history. Cattle, sheep, and goats graze, and pigs and poultry manage on wild plants and scraps — pretty much the type of win-win situation outlined at the start of this chapter. But even these systems only remain sustainable if the animals are kept in low densities per unit of land and within the capacity of the specific environment.

The reality, however, is that in many parts of the world, livestock are too numerous for their ecosystems. In the case of ruminants, they're often overgrazed. Especially in developing countries, they often roam in such numbers and on land so dry and bare that it eventually degrades into desert. Such practices occur for many reasons including rising human population, lack of access to productive land for the poor, and policy frameworks that "often exacerbate livestock's impact on

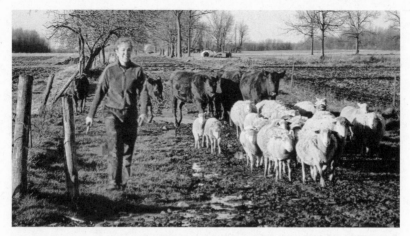

Livestock is integrated naturally into crop production on this organic mixed farm in southern Ontario run by farmer-activist Colleen Ross and her family. You'll meet Ms. Ross later in the book.

the environment," according to the FAO.[63] These frameworks include national and international objectives for large-scale production (discussed later in this book) and specific rules and regulations that can actually discourage efficient use of land, water, and other resources.[64]

But subsistence farmers in sub-Saharan Africa are not the problem. Far from discouraging animal husbandry, the FAO has a "pro-poor livestock" policy in the developing world, aimed at poverty alleviation,[65] and it also works to help farmers lessen Livestock's Long Shadow. Nor is anyone suggesting that all global citizens cut back on their livestock holdings, or eat less meat. We in industrialized countries need to take the lead on lowering the environmental impact of meat—based simply on equity and access to alternatives. Most of us in wealthy countries eat far more meat than do citizens of developing countries. Most of us already take in enough calories without large amounts of flesh foods. Most of us have ready access to plant-based foods and meat alternatives. And most of us can locate citizen organizations, elected officials, and food manufacturers through whom we can encourage sustainable production.

This responsibility especially applies to those of us in cities who are pure consumers when it comes to animal products, and indeed to most foods.[66] Unlike rural residents, who are producers as well as consumers of meat and milk, we who live in condos and neighborhoods are not givers but takers. This gives us extra responsibility for not taking more than our environmental share.

Taking the lead will include a combination of measures to improve the way we make and eat animal-source foods. There's no shortage of possibilities on the production side (which I detail in later chapters). For example, if livestock diets are tweaked in specific ways, ruminants produce less methane. If land is managed with low-till and other conservation tactics, more carbon is sequestered in the soil. If manure is stored with more attention to physical containment and temperature control, fewer gases arise.

But all the methodological production efficiencies in the world are unlikely to solve the meat problem. As discussed more in Chapter 6, if we're going to lower agricultural greenhouse gas emissions to sustainable levels, heavy consumers will need to trim back.

Convincing people to keep their intake to sustainable levels won't be easy. But one intriguing suggestion has been offered by a group of scientists headed by Australian epidemiologist Anthony McMichael. In a widely quoted article published in the medical journal *The Lancet*,[67] the group calls for international discussions and negotiated agreements to set target levels of sustainable production and consumption.

Termed a "contraction and convergence" strategy (after the climate-change concept), the plan would require high-consumption countries to contract their intake downward, while low-consumption countries would (in some cases) be able to expand their meat intake. Eventually all parties would converge on some agreed-upon level that the planet could sustain. Needless to say, consumers in the United States and Canada would be asked to make bigger concessions than would consumers in most other parts of the world. I'll give you the numbers in Chapter 6, but here I'll simply say that, under a plan like this, we in wealthy countries may need to cut our consumption by more than half.

The idea of contraction and convergence has gained attention internationally, and it has been promoted by groups including Compassion in World Farming in the UK as part of a "Vision for Fair Food and

Farming." That vision supports "reduced consumption of animal products in high-consuming populations to meet environmental, health and sustainability goals."[68]

Whatever the specific strategies, we can find ways to address the serious problems for land and climate that stem from too many livestock. We can improve production, and we can reduce consumption. A pile of reports shows that many scientists agree.[69] Keeping livestock can be practiced sustainably, if it is done in lower densities and under more natural conditions that are sensible for healthy ecosystems.

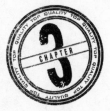

Water is Being Used and Abused

Activists Are Testing the Waters

Larry Baldwin towers over the grassy ledge and stretches down toward the streambed to fill a beaker with water. He and his team of environmental advocates have parked their trucks just down the road from a factory pig farm here in eastern North Carolina. They're on public property, and the water-quality testing they're doing is not only legal but in the public interest — part of their work to monitor the streams and tributaries that make up the Neuse River. But the factory farm operators don't like it, and today one of them has driven over in his pickup and is standing in dark sunglasses, arms folded, making sure they know he's there.

Being observed is part of the job when you're a Neuse Riverkeeper and an employee of the international Waterkeeper Alliance,[1] the watchdog group led by environmentalist Robert F. Kennedy, Jr. On one occasion, Mr. Baldwin was confronted by factory farm staff with guns on their dashboards, so he won't let volunteers do any sampling alone. On this day, I'm new and nervous. But the team persists, retrieving samples and recording information on exact location, water temperature, and other details — carefully, in case the data need to stand up in court. Later, as the rest of us drive back to the nearby town of New Bern,

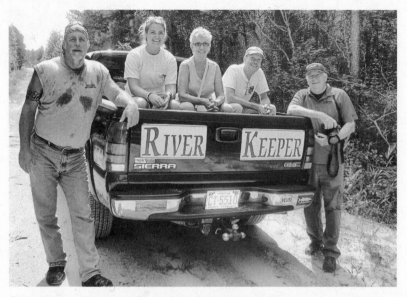

Clean-water advocates after a day of sampling in streams near intensive livestock operations in North Carolina. L to R: Larry Baldwin, Kelsey Hansen, Joanne Somerday, John Klecker, Rick Dove.

Mr. Baldwin drops off the samples at the lab where technicians will test for fecal coliform, ammonia, nitrates, phosphorus, and other pollutants. If pollutants are detected, the test results can be used to charge polluters under the federal Clean Water Act.

One of the major rivers in North Carolina, the Neuse is a gorgeous network of streams and tributaries that snake through the land. With a long history of providing food and livelihoods to residents, the Neuse is home to fish and other aquatic life. But the river has been polluted in recent decades — enough to kill what both environmentalists and scientists calculate as over one billion fish.[2] That's not million, but billion. Rick Dove, former Riverkeeper and a key figure in the group, has witnessed these mass die-offs, including the 1991 event when environmentalists say hundreds of millions of dead fish turned up.[3] Mr. Dove showed me photographic evidence on his website. You look at the images of fish with gaping holes in their bodies, he observes, and you say it can't be true. But it's documented in academic and government studies — dead fish in what should be a clean and healthy river.[4]

A major pollution challenge here is visible from the air. We flew over Duplin County to see the highest concentration of intensive hog farms in the United States, in a state that has 9.5 million people but 10 million hogs. We witnessed factory farms as far as we could see — row upon row of long buildings, each packed with thousands of animals. And beside these farms were pools of feces and urine the size of football fields.[5] Officially called "lagoons" in the livestock business, they also go by less flattering names. I've read scientific articles on these potent pools and heard the evidence that their contents can leak into soil, contaminate groundwater, and emit toxic gases. Here in eastern North Carolina, many CAFOs were built in the late 1980s, and since the lagoons are thought to have lifespan of only a few decades,[6] environmentalists expect breaches and breakdowns soon. Breaches are especially likely during the frequent rain or storms in the region. Seepages into groundwater are also more likely here than in some parts of the country, because in eastern North Carolina there's a relatively small amount of soil between the bottom of a lagoon and the water table below.[7]

Massive chicken barns, an increasing trend, are also visible from the air. We banked and circled over one chicken facility and a nearby waste pile adjacent to a stream. "The environmental legislation is weak," commented one of my flying companions. And what there is isn't always enforced, he added. As we fly, we see operators spraying manure onto fields that are brown from drought. The job appears to be not just fertilization, but also waste disposal.

Companies that own these intensive operations claim the manure is good fertilizer and they carefully apply it in amounts appropriate to croplands. They say factory farm operators adhere to nutrient management plans and safely manage their waste.[8] But while operators may be following rules, and consumers may be getting their meat, scientists who study the river say it is contaminated from manure. According to biologist JoAnn Burkholder: "The major source of pollution to the lower Neuse watershed/estuary is swine CAFOs."[9] Director of the Center for Applied Aquatic Ecology at North Carolina State University, Dr. Burkholder has actively studied the Neuse for more than 20 years. She oversees a long-term research and monitoring program there and has published extensively on the topic.[10] Since the 1980s, the entire river has been classified as "nutrient sensitive," she told me, meaning it has algae blooms, oxygen deficiencies, and major fish kills. Some attempt has been made to clean up the river, and some crop farmers deserve praise, as do several cities that have installed better waste treatment systems. But "the swine CAFO industry has done very little to reduce its massive pollution," according to Dr. Burkholder. Hog production, plus intensive poultry, plus ever more people and industry, all produce too much waste.

Water quality in the Neuse is, in some ways, getting worse, says Dr. Burkholder. Ammonium levels rose by 500% between 1994 and 2003.[11] Ammonium increases the amounts of toxic or otherwise noxious algae, which thrive on it and fuel eutrophication — a process whereby excess chemicals such as phosphates and nitrates act as fertilizers and stimulate overgrowth of vegetation that chokes out other plants and fish. Sediment at the bottom of the river is so contaminated that the estuary can no longer support the food web for its historically high levels of striped bass and other desirable fish species.[12]

Water testing provides scientific information to document pollution. But water activists are also testing the waters in a legal sense. In a case now before the courts in Maryland, Waterkeeper Alliance is suing not only the day-to-day operators of a factory farm they claim is contaminating local waters, but also the corporation that owns the farm.[13] To date, corporations have been able to claim that they don't own the livestock waste, under contracts with the growers, who run the daily operations. A successful challenge would be precedent-setting, says water activist Kathy Phillips, official Coastkeeper on the Maryland shore.[14] According to Phillips, broiler chicken manure is deposited on crop fields and some ends up in waterways — and companies wash their hands of it. "Every single aspect of a broiler's life is controlled by the corporation, and yet somehow when the chicken poops, at some point between the chicken butt and the ground, that poop magically becomes the responsibility of the grower and not the owner of the chicken."[15] Lawyer Hannah Connor, who has worked for Waterkeepers, agrees that corporations should share any blame for pollution, that "the liability should be spread across the parties," and that the case could have dramatic implications in making agribusiness responsible for waste.[16]

Livestock are by no means the sole source of pollution on the river. On the upper Neuse, contaminants also come from urbanization and human sewage treatment plants.[17] On the lower Neuse, sources include wastewater facilities, septic tanks, car exhaust, crop fertilizers, and atmospheric deposition. But even this latter is to some degree from swine production, and adding to it in the lower Neuse is manure and other waste from the many CAFOs in the region.

This is not a healthy waterway, observes Rick Dove back at the Riverkeeper office in New Bern. So many animals, so much fecal matter laying open for months, cooking in the summer sun and getting whipped up by weather. "And there's no way they can spray that much hog waste on land here without contaminating the river." It begs larger questions, he says. "When you violate all of these natural laws, at some point there are consequences." If we continue with current methods of animal agriculture, some ecological or public health crisis could hit. Yet there is action we can take. We can change the way livestock are produced.

Waste Is Not a Pretty Topic

Fortunately for the meat business, no one likes to talk about biological waste. Our natural aversion is strong; as one book aptly puts it, this waste is *The Last Taboo*.[18] Often alluded to by scientists and government officials as "water problems," manure is discussed in the livestock industry as almost synonymous with "nutrients."[19] Indeed, livestock waste should be nutrient fertilizer, and in small amounts, from low-density agricultural systems, it is. But in excess, it is called by other names. One 2005 Manitoba group concerned about pathogenic levels of manure fertilizers labeled itself Citizens for the Responsible Application of Phosphorus, with an acronym that spoke for itself.

Agribusiness terminology includes "lagoons" for the pools of feces and urine outside intensive operations.[20] Don Webb, a 70-something North Carolinian who has been fighting factory farms for years, has something to say about that. "They call those places lagoons," he told me. "Well, to me a lagoon is a pool of water on a South Seas Island where a beautiful woman swims. These factory farm manure pits aren't lagoons. They're cesspools."[21] In this opinion, Mr. Webb is not alone. A report from the Natural Resources Defense Council on pollution from factory farms was called "Cesspools of Shame."[22]

Walkerton, Ontario, provides a striking example of our reluctance to talk about what's behind water pollution. This small Canadian community made big news in 2000 when thousands of residents fell ill after brushing their teeth, drinking tap water, and routinely using this everyday resource. Many of the ill landed in hospital, and seven people died.

Why was the water so polluted? What caused the disease outbreak? Investigators cited a list of factors.[23] Regulatory procedures were lax. Purification systems were inadequate. And water monitoring was incompetent, for which two officials took the blame. But important as such factors are to good government, they aren't very helpful to us as citizens. You and I have no direct control over water-quality systems, and we know that human error sometimes occurs. It makes us feel there's little we can do. So let's ask how the town's water got dirty in the first place, and why so many of our water supplies need to be tested and treated, screened, and scrubbed. At the risk of sounding naïve, why do we need laws, regulations, and powerful chemicals to keep our water clean? What's behind Walkerton is what's behind a lot of problems for the environment and public health.

It was no secret that the actual disease-causing pathogens came from cattle manure. That was spelled out in the official investigative report from Medical Health Officer Dr. Murray McQuigge, and it was reiterated in the findings of the provincial inquiry led by Supreme Court Justice Dennis O'Connor. Located in a region with a high density of livestock, Walkerton is surrounded by meat and dairy production. Thirteen livestock farms within a mere 4 km radius of the town's contaminated water wells were geographically positioned in a way that resulted in some risk of runoff toward one or more of the wells.[24] As the report stated, the virulent bacteria came from cattle from at least one of these farms, whose herd later tested positive for the strain of E. coli O157.H7 that factored into the illness and death.

It wasn't the farmers' fault. The provincial inquiry cited a specific agricultural operation that was the probable contamination source and said: "The owner of this farm followed proper practices and should not be faulted."[25] At least the events prompted improvements to what is considered good practice by all parties. Prior to Walkerton, waste management guidelines asked for voluntary compliance, says Sarah Miller, coordinator and researcher at the Canadian Environmental Law Association. "After Walkerton, the association worked hard to secure several new laws for safe drinking water, protection of the sources of drinking water, and regulating improved manure management."[26] In the future, especially given the trend to extreme weather events,[27] more jurisdictions may need stricter regulatory systems.

Yet regulatory systems weren't the original source of the manure. It came from too many livestock animals in too small a geographical region — all to satisfy meat-centered food systems and eating habits. There is more than simply embarrassment that keeps us from discussing livestock manure. When large amounts of meat are being produced by powerful sectors of the economy to feed widespread consumer expectations, there is little motivation for officials to address the fundamental subject. However, the problem can motivate us as citizens to question our habit of eating meat and dairy products in quantity every day. It's not a pretty topic, but we may not have the luxury of avoiding manure if we're going to address the problems of livestock and meat.

This Much Manure Isn't Fertilizer, It's Pollution

Excellent fertilizer is what manure can be, and in small quantities it is. But tens of billions of livestock produce waste that in some cases and places is simply too much. As has been said about finances: "Money is like manure, of very little use except it be spread," which interestingly was coined by the 16th-century philosopher Francis Bacon.

Even in unnatural environments like intensive livestock facilities, nature calls daily. And when animals answer the call, they excrete heaps. It's impossible to calculate the amounts of manure produced, not only from factory farms but from the hundreds of millions of animals that let it drop on fields. Exactly how much manure there is depends on what you're measuring, but the numbers are sobering. The comprehensive Pew Commission report on factory farming said that the animals confined in US CAFOs produce three times as much manure as the human sewage produced in the country as a whole.[28] But if you're just counting biosolids (the heavy parts that settle out), animal feeding operations in the United States produce 100 times as much as municipal wastewater plants have of the human stuff.[29] I found that statistic so alarming that I checked it out with the lead scientist on the report, Charles Gerba, at the University of Arizona, who confirmed the numbers. An environmental microbiologist, Dr. Gerba has written extensively on pollution and has said that large-scale livestock waste used as crop fertilizer can be a health hazard. Dairy cattle are especially prolific, with one cow producing waste equal to that of 20–40 people, according to the US EPA.[30]

All this livestock output doesn't get much treatment, which industry says is reasonable because animal waste — unlike the human variant — is allowable and desirable fertilizer. Whether leavings from livestock get any treatment depends on your point of view. Some environmentalists claim it gets none, and it does get less treatment than the flushings from our toilets, even though the voluminous output of cattle, pigs, and chickens can contain veterinary drugs, vaccines, growth hormones, disinfectants, and disease agents.[31]

But the CAFO system of storing waste in lagoons does allow solids to settle out, and it allows naturally occurring bacteria to biologically reduce the inherent carbon load, so it does qualify as primary treatment in the view of Mike Williams, a professor at North Carolina State University and director of their Animal and Poultry Waste Management Center.[32] Dr. Williams does not agree with critics who say water pollution from livestock production is at a crisis point. But he does call current management of hog manure unsustainable for the long term.[33] Dr. Williams is not endorsing prevailing methods. Superior waste management systems do exist and should be used, he says. He headed a research team that spent years evaluating alternative systems for managing CAFO manure, ultimately identifying and publicizing five alternative technologies.[34] But as we'll see in Chapter 6, not many producers have signed on.

Livestock manure needs proper management partly because it contains a lot of chemical compounds. Animals are not very efficient digesters when fed unnatural diets, like the corn and grain fed to ruminants. So their manure contains large amounts of unmetabolized carbohydrates, fats, and sugars, as well as the microorganisms that arise and spread in their irritated digestive tracts. Waste also contains large amounts of plant and animal drugs and chemicals from fertilizers that were applied to feed. Unfortunately, much of what they take in they excrete right out the other end. A productive dairy cow can release most of the nitrogen, phosphorus, and other chemicals it has ingested.[35]

Manure should be spread. But given the number of animals in factory farms and the amount of manure they create, there is often too little land to put it on. Nearby crop fields often can't accommodate the volumes, and trucking large amounts of manure around the countryside can be too costly and labor-intensive. So, agricultural lands get saddled with more than they can handle. Then all you need is one good rain for manure to flow into the nearest stream.

Water has long been used by humans for waste disposal. Lake Winnipeg, on the Canadian Prairies, is so large that it should be able to take some such abuse, and a local politician there was known for declaring that "the solution to pollution is dilution."[36] But the waste is so plentiful that it is difficult to dilute, even in the tenth largest freshwater lake in the world, larger than the state of Vermont. A natural wonder, Lake Winnipeg is a focal point for life, work, and recreation in Manitoba. Nevertheless, one report after another has indicated that the water is dirty. It is also surrounded by hogs. There are twice as many of these large pigs as humans in the province — 2.6 million animals in mid-2010 compared with 1.2 million people. Eight million pigs were produced there during 2010,[37] many in animal factories near Lake Winnipeg or adjoining waterways.

Hogs have been controversial in Manitoba for years. But as a large agricultural business, the basis of a major food-processing industry, and a significant export product, hogs are good for the bottom line. Yet the evidence is strong that Manitoba hog production adds to water pollution. It's been laid out in years of scientific reports, including a 2007 publication from the province's Clean Environment Commission.[38] The Commission held months of hearings and received hundreds of submissions and presentations to conclude that steps needed to be taken for the future industry to be sustainable. There is too much waste and chemicals for Manitoba's water systems, said the report. Livestock producers spread excessive manure on soils, and, notes the Commission, the provincial government is aware of the situation.[39] The spreading continues in spite of the evidence that hog waste is particularly polluting, with a biochemical oxygen demand considerably higher than municipal human sewage.[40] That means hog waste removes inordinate amounts of oxygen from water, accelerating the process of eutrophication that can suffocate fish and natural plants.

Eva Pip is a Winnipeg scientist who has criticized the hog industry for pollution. A professor of biology at the University of Winnipeg and an expert on water quality, she's one of those people who has decided it's more important to speak out than to be popular. "If you say anything against intensive livestock operations, you're considered to be anti-jobs and anti-business," said Dr. Pip in an interview with me. So most government officials and even some scientists, she says, are reluctant to discuss large-scale hog production as a contributor to the degradation of Lake Winnipeg.[41]

When I visited Dr. Pip's university lab, she talked about the evidence. She and her students have done rigorous sampling. They've found dangerous toxins in the lake and measured the potentially lethal substance "microcystin" at sometimes 400 times the allowable limit for human health. Local beaches were closed at the height of the problem, but that's no solution to pollution. The lake is burdened with discharge from the city, from lake cottages, and from other industry. But hog waste is prolific.

It's no coincidence that intensive livestock operations affect waterways; it's convenient for them to be located near rivers and lakes so they can meet their water needs. Manitoba hog barns are often sited near

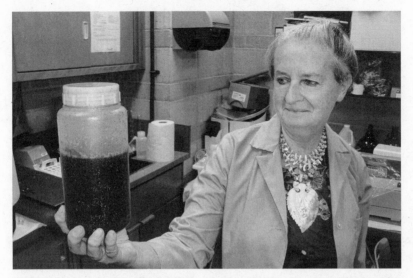

Biology professor Dr. Eva Pip, with a sample of contaminated water from Lake Winnipeg. Pollution to the lake comes partly from the millions of hogs produced around the lake and its nearby waterways.

water, and Dr. Pip has demonstrated that surface and ground supplies can subsequently become polluted downstream.[42]

Life isn't easy for investigators who raise these issues. But Dr. Pip persists, and she wrote a detailed scientific critique of the intensive live-stock industry for the government.[43] One activist told me Dr. Pip has been severely criticized for warning of potential pollution and being an environmental advocate, but "her predictions have unfortunately come to fruition."[44]

Industry takes a different point of view, contending that hogs are only a minor source of pollution that contribute but a small percentage of the contaminants to Lake Winnipeg.[45] The Manitoba Pork Council in 2011 published a report "Embracing a Sustainable Future," which de-fended the pork business as good for jobs and good for production — not only of pork, but of other consumer products. The report laid out 82 commitments from the industry to make, or to keep, hog production environmentally viable for the long term.[46]

Producers are indeed aware of the issues and are making improve-ments. But some observers say the system needs an overhaul and that no major strides will be taken without policies supporting a new kind of livestock production. The Canadian citizen group Beyond Factory Farming[47] promotes what it calls "socially responsible livestock," campaigns against factory farm pollution, and seeks tighter environmental regulations and far-reaching changes to the way we raise animals. The group thinks we're more likely to get socially responsible systems if we recognize two principles of ecology: (1) Everything is connected to everything else; and (2) There is no free lunch.[48] Intensive livestock operations are connected to everything else in their ecosystems. And our "free lunch" of inexpensive meat is exacting a cost on the environment and our health.

> "The livestock sector is a key player in increasing water use....It is probably the largest sectoral source of water pollution, contributing to eutrophication, 'dead zones' in coastal areas, degradation of coral reefs, human health problems, emergence of antibiotic resistance and many others. The main sources of pollution are from animal wastes, antibiotics and hormones, chemicals from tanneries, fertilizers and pesticides used for feedcrops, and sediments from eroded pastures."
>
> — Steinfeld et al., *Livestock's Long Shadow*, UN Food and Agriculture Organization, 2006, p. xxiii.

Water Around the World Is Getting Wasted

"Probably the largest sectoral source of water pollution." That's how the FAO assesses global livestock production.[49] In some parts of Asia, home to large and growing meat factories, pig waste is now a bigger polluter than is human domestic waste.[50] There are many other examples internationally and at home. In the United States and Canada, contamination from manure is common. Waterways in Iowa have been fouled by intensively raised swine and other animals.[51] Rivers in southern Ontario should provide clean swimming beaches, but are polluted from animal and other agriculture, says Mark Mattson, the Toronto-based Lake Ontario waterkeeper.[52] In Alberta's Feedlot Alley, 300 square miles of cattle production just north of Montana, scientists have found "continually high populations of E. coli,"[53] along with health-threatening amounts of bacteria in area waters.[54] It's hard to stop so much livestock from leaving some of their leavings behind.

The Lower Fraser Valley is lush and lovely where it stretches east from Vancouver, British Columbia. But its underground aquifers are polluted, in part by the 50–75 million intensively raised chickens produced there each year.[55] The industry brings forth a lot of food, but also a lot of manure. Because there's more than what nearby crops can use, some of it "will eventually end up in receiving waters," says international water expert Hans Schreier.[56] The underground aquifer there should be a good source of drinking water, but it contains high levels of pathogenic compounds. Many wells in the area "have levels of nitrate well above the national drinking water guidelines."[57] Faculty member at the University of British Columbia's Institute for Resources, Environment and Sustainability, Dr. Schreier says there are too many animals in too little space. The Lower Fraser Valley has the highest livestock density in Canada, with more farm animals per square unit of land (mostly chickens) than anywhere else in the country. It also has the highest concentration of factory farms. In much of this region, animal-stocking densities are almost twice what is allowed in Denmark, where a long history of animal agriculture — plus more people per square mile, plus deeper citizen awareness of environmental issues — motivates policy-makers toward systems that will be viable long term. Dr. Schreier believes water policy in British Columbia and elsewhere needs to limit livestock densities, improve manure management, and enforce water-quality guidelines.[58]

Around the world, there are countless stories of compromised water. As marine dead zones proliferate, many shoreline regions have too little oxygen to support normal aquatic life. Try an Internet search for "dead zones" and you'll find disturbing documentation of this sorry situation, including global maps from NASA showing numerous dead zones along the Atlantic coast.[59] One of the world's most formidable dead zones is in the Gulf of Mexico, at the mouth of the Mississippi River — it's due largely to excess fertilizers and manure, much of which can be traced directly or indirectly to intensive livestock farming.[60]

Sufficient and Clean Water Should Be Priorities

Humans use a lot of freshwater. We drink it and boil potatoes in it. We take showers, wash our clothes and cars, flush our toilets, and water our lawns. But those activities account for only a small portion of human water use. I was raised to be cautious in consumption, and am uncomfortable when others leave a kitchen tap running or take long showers. But that's not really the main problem.

As much as 70% of human-used freshwater is used for agriculture, and much of that goes to raise animals for meat and dairy products.[61] Such water use might be tolerable if it were necessary to feed humans well. But since the evidence suggests we're eating too many animal products for our health or the environment, it's hard to justify continuing to ramp up production of foods that use disproportionate amounts of this necessity of life.

"Meat is by far the most water-consumptive food," says Hans Schreier. Staples like grain and rice require 1,000–2,000 liters of water to make a kilogram of food, while beef requires more than 15,000 liters to make a kilogram of meat.[62] Overall, producing meat requires at least ten times as much water as producing the same amount of grain, fruit, or vegetables.[63] Some calculations reveal even greater differentials. Because of this, heavy meat-eaters implicitly use much more water than do vegetarians or light-to-moderate meat-eaters. Water use is particularly intensive in dairy production. And because meat and dairy intake are increasing rapidly, livestock-related water use is projected to jump 50% by 2025.[64]

Meanwhile, the world is water-stressed. Those of us who live near oceans may feel we're swimming in it. But that's saltwater, as is over 95% of the globe's water supply. Freshwater, essential to life, constitutes only a few percent of planetary liquid, and much of it is locked up in glaciers and the atmosphere. Shortages are worldwide. Droughts are widespread and increasingly common, undermining agriculture from the southern US states to the Horn of Africa. Water tables are falling in almost every country that irrigates from underground.[65] Throughout the US Great Plains, wells have gone dry, forcing farmers to revert to lower-yield dryland farming. In India, China, and many other nations, agriculture is taking more water than can naturally be replenished. "Suddenly it is so clear: the world is running out of fresh water," say Maude Barlow and Tony Clarke, authors of the book *Blue Gold* on global problems and skirmishes over water.[66]

Livestock animals are thirsty creatures, and they need their species-specific versions of eight glasses a day. Large cattle can each drink many gallons a day. Studies on "virtual water," calculating the volumes required to produce a commodity, show that when you include what's used to produce the animals' feed, it can take a striking 200–250 gallons of water to create a single gallon of milk.[67] Raising small animals for food doesn't use as much, but any kind of meat requires more liquid input than the same amount of plant food, whether measured in calories, proteins, or fats.[68]

Even traditional livestock systems stress water resources when there are too many animals on the range. Excessive cattle or goats chew vegetation down to the dirt, destabilizing soil that then becomes unable to hold water. High densities of animals can trample the ground and interfere with natural ecosystems. Valuable topsoil blows away, and deserts spread. This has already happened in many overgrazed regions on the planet.

But water use is especially high on factory farms, where not only do cattle, pigs, and chickens get thirsty, but water is required for "servicing," which includes cleaning production areas, washing out barns, washing and cooling animals, and disposing of the urine and feces.[69]

I mentioned above that feed production is partly responsible for meaty water use, and let me emphasize this. Though most of us rarely think about feed crops, the fact is that the most substantial use of water for intensive livestock is for growing soy, corn, barley, and the like for fattening the animals. Of all water used to make all foods around the world, livestock takes almost half, and that's mostly to grow feed for factory farms. Producing feed uses almost 90% of the water that goes into meat and dairy products.[70] All that liquid for feed crops rarely gets counted in official estimates of livestock-related water use, according to the FAO. In many jurisdictions, policymakers reckon only the water actually used on livestock farms, which is a "considerable underestimate"[71] of total water use and depletion for making meat and milk.

Protecting our water should be at the top of every government's agenda. But the state of many of our waterways suggests it is not. Most citizens aren't aware that our water is in trouble, both in quantity and quality, or that large-scale livestock production plays a role. Policymakers themselves aren't always informed. "The impacts of the livestock sector on water resources are often not well understood by decision-makers,"[72] says *Livestock's Long Shadow.* In the United States, Canada, and elsewhere, many jurisdictions have inadequate laws and regulations to protect water from exhaustion and pollution. Where laws exist, they are often loosely enforced. As the FAO observes: "In developed countries, regulatory frameworks exist, but rules are often circumvented or violated."[73] As a result, livestock around the world have compromised water through overuse and contamination.

For those of us who turn on the tap each day and get cups full of drinkable water, it's hard to imagine that many millions of our international neighbors cannot.[74] Meanwhile, many of us consume daily portions of some of the thirstiest foods on Earth.

Livestock production could be done better. Meat could be made using less water and causing less pollution, even within current production models, with more efficient feed crop irrigation, land management techniques such as rotational grazing, and better management of waste. Meat could be made even more ecologically under new models relying on lower-density livestock systems and more natural feeding and waste management protocols. Making this happen will require visionary public policy.[75] We citizens can encourage such policy, and at the consumer level can conserve water and minimize pollution by eating lower on the food chain, consuming fewer water-consumptive foods, and supporting the best kinds of sustainable livestock producers.

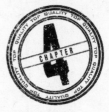

TOO MUCH MEAT ADDS TO ILLNESS AND DISEASE

Moderation Is a Prescription for Health

Avian and swine flus, antibiotic-resistant infections, mad cow disease, heart conditions, and cancers. It sounds like the index from a medical textbook, but it is actually a list of just some of the many health problems connected to large-scale meat production or consumption. Every one of these illnesses is multifactorial, with contributions from many different sources. But each one can be exacerbated by mass production of livestock or heavy consumption of meat. Producing too much meat, especially in confined animal feeding operations (CAFOs), exposes communities to large amounts of manure, antibiotics, and other drugs, as well as fertilizers and pesticides from feed crops. Once the meat is made, eating too much of it increases our vulnerability to a range of chronic medical conditions including obesity, cardiovascular disease, and diabetes.[1]

It's all about moderation. If an occasional glass of wine adds to health and happiness, that doesn't mean you should sit down and polish off the bottle. It's the same with animal products. If a little is good, it doesn't follow that a lot is better. Raising and eating less meat would probably lead to better health — for us, for the livestock, and for the environment.

Even food safety crises that get blamed on vegetables can be connected to excessive meat production. Food-related illnesses from the bacteria *E. coli* are often in the news, sometimes leaving us with the impression that vegetables are dangerous and that maybe we should stop eating leafy greens or sprouts. You may remember the 2006 "spinach outbreak" of *E. coli* O157:H7 in California that sickened more than 200 people and caused three deaths.[2] But *E. coli* is a product not of vegetables, but of animals.[3] Normally found in the intestines of warm-blooded creatures, "*E. coli* does not usually occur naturally on plants or in soil or water," says Health Canada.[4] In the case of the tainted spinach, an investigation by the FDA and state authorities did not identify the exact means by which bacteria spread to the spinach, but one possible source was "surface waterways exposed to feces from cattle and wild-life."[5] It's true that there were some wild boar in the area. But there were also a lot of cattle.[6] Given the sheer population of livestock animals today, all of which are producing waste — much of which is used in large amounts on crops and then washed into waterways — the real culprit may be too much manure. We still need more research to know how often livestock waste figures in food safety crises. While waiting for that, however, rather than eat fewer vegetables, we might ease back on animal-source foods so these can be made in modest amounts, creating limited waste that is within the capacity of the planet to absorb.

The health downsides of high-volume meat production are illustrated by a seemingly small example — the state of the air inside factory farms. The air is often heavily laden with particles. It can contain dust from feed and bedding materials, bits of dried dung and urine, feathers and hair, chemicals, and bacteria. In outdoor environments, these would be diluted in the ambient atmosphere.[7] But to breathe inside a factory farm is to risk inhaling these particles as well as airborne ammonia, hydrogen sulfide, and methane. Factory farms can contribute to respiratory maladies, chronic fatigue, and other syndromes in pigs, cattle, chickens, and humans.[8] Employees, despite masks and other protective gear, often suffer unpleasant physiological responses, as do the animals.[9]

But the atmosphere of factory farms can affect even those who never step inside. When you drive through CAFO country, you see animal factories with giant circular wall fans used to expel the air. And that means neighbors are in for it, too. CAFO-area residents are more likely than others to suffer not only physical problems involving the lungs, sinuses, and digestive system, but mental problems as well.[10] People who live near large hog factories are more prone to respiratory and digestive illnesses, along with headaches, sore throats, and diarrhoea.[11] On the Canadian Prairies, if you live near a feedlot, you're more likely to show symptoms of intestinal, respiratory, and other diseases.[12] We're even imposing this air on children; odors can be noticed both outside and inside area schools, and young people living closer to CAFOs tend to show more symptoms of allergies.[13]

The smell around factory farms is not the pleasant rural scent of new harvest, good fresh dirt, and a whiff of waste. Having driven through intensive livestock regions, I can attest that the experience can assault the senses. Just breathing in and out can bring on coughing fits. The stench of factory farms has become a major community issue in countrysides in the United States, Canada, and elsewhere. The odor and pollution add to neighbors' tension, depression, anger, confusion, and fatigue,[14] leaving many with a diminished feeling of having control over their lives.[15] One Manitoba report claimed that a hog industry supporter taunted rural residents who dared complain.[16] "If you want fresh air," he said, "move to the city."

Air should be fresh. It should also be invisible. But as long as meat production is invisible to most of us — with its animals and methods locked behind closed doors — it will have the potential to compromise our health.

Factory Farming Fuels Animal-to-Human Diseases

So many animals have been killed in recent years to stop avian and other animal flus, that most of us have lost track. In 1997 in Hong Kong, an outbreak of H5N1 avian flu caused such panic that the entire poultry population of about 1.5 million birds was killed within a few days.[17]

In the Fraser Valley near Vancouver, 13 million or more poultry were killed in 2004 to contain bird flu.[18] In just the past few years, hundreds of millions of birds globally have either been killed by bird flu, or been culled to stop its spread.[19] Foot-and-mouth disease among livestock in Britain sparked a cull of as many as 10 million animals in 2001.[20] It's been all over the news: details of wasted animal lives, wasted time and investment from farmers, and wasted human food.

Zoonose, or *zoonosis*, is the scientific term for an illness humans can catch from animals, including bird flu, swine flu, and diseases with acronyms like BSE, FMD, and SARS.[21] Pronounced "zo-oh-noze" and "zo-oh-nosis," such diseases are sometimes labeled pandemics, though not all are sufficiently widespread to get that designation from the World Health Organization. Nevertheless, animal-to-human diseases are worrisome. They make up most of new pathologies today, and though some are benign, others are not.[22] At a recent international conference devoted to zoonoses, organizers warned that recent events have shown humans to be "very vulnerable."[23]

It is difficult to talk about these phenomena without sounding alarmist, but one or more could cause widespread health crises. Modern animal viruses can mutate and adapt quickly, and humans don't have much immunity to them. Some affect mostly livestock, not humans, but viruses and bacteria are clever survivors, and they find ways to infect new hosts. They also have increasing numbers of environments in which to flourish and multiply, including factory farms.

Swine flu hit the headlines when this previously benign animal virus became dangerous to people. Like a lot of pathogens, this one had been around for years. It was a common virus, but it had been stable, causing mostly manageable cases of respiratory disease in pigs. But over time, there were signs that the virus was becoming more contagious.[24] It showed itself in the spring of 2009 in residents living near large-scale industrial pig operations in the Mexican state of Veracruz.[25] People there had been complaining about the pig production, its smell and manure, and their infections and respiratory problems. By mid-June, more than 100 people in Mexico had died from the virus H1N1 that came to be known as swine flu.[26] The first American, a Texas schoolteacher, succumbed in May of that year.[27] Representatives of the Mexican pig factory claimed there was no swine flu, but when you raise about a million pigs a year in close quarters, keeping them healthy is hard to do.[28]

Scientific analyses showed the H1N1 swine flu to be a new combination of viruses that was more aggressive and dangerous than its components or predecessor strains. The World Health Organization declared it a pandemic, and over the next year, cases were confirmed in more than 200 countries and territories. Since then, human deaths worldwide from the swine flu have totaled more than 18,000.[29]

What bothers Cathy Holtslander is that people blame the pigs. A long-time environmental advocate with the citizen group Beyond Factory Farming, she believes such diseases are caused not by animals, but by the intensive methods by which we raise them.[30] Too many animals in too small a space facilitates disease. Michael Greger, a physician, agricultural writer, and expert on bird flus, says animal factories bear some resemblance to medieval cities, where overcrowding and lack of sanitation led to all kinds of disease.[31] In the words of GRAIN, an international non-governmental organization for sustainable agriculture, "Experts have been warning for years that the rise of large-scale factory farms in North America has created the perfect breeding grounds for the emergence and spread of new highly-virulent strains of influenza."[32]

We don't need to be scientists to imagine how industrial meat production promotes zoonoses. First, the animals are crowded, making it more likely for pathogens to jump from one chicken or pig to another. Second, the air inside factory farms contains dust, waste, and fumes. Third, the animals are genetically similar or even identical, lacking the biological diversity that helps protect against disease.[33] Fourth, the animals are stressed — they are often prevented from engaging in natural activities such as caring for their young, moving around to find food, or even interacting with one another, and they are sometimes subjected to painful procedures without anesthetic.[34]

In the old days, new or so-called novel pathogens would be geographically confined. But along with intensive production comes rising international trade in meat.[35] Live animals, body parts, and meat and livestock feed are trucked, shipped, and flown around the globe — in increasing quantities each decade. Though it may contradict ecological common sense, it is not unusual for pigs to be born in North Carolina, fattened in the Corn Belt of Iowa, and slaughtered in California. Even more dramatically, more than a billion live animals are moved across borders each year.[36]

Not only animal mobility, but also human mobility, adds to the spread of zoonoses. This was illustrated with the rise of SARS (severe acute respiratory syndrome), the viral flu that appears to have crossed the species barrier from exotic food animals to humans in Chinese street markets in early 2003. The species involved included small mammals called civets, which have the misfortune to be the subject of a belief that consumption of their penises will boost the sex drive.[37] One man picked up the virus, then attended a wedding in Hong Kong, where he presumably coughed on others. As guests departed for their far-flung homes, they took the virus to five countries within 24 hours, sparking a process that caused hundreds of human deaths.[38]

Bovine spongiform encephalopathy (BSE) is another worrisome animal-to-human illness. Also called mad cow disease, it causes neural tissue to disintegrate in cow brains. The human variant of the disease is called Creutzfeldt-Jakob disease (vCJD). It is passed on to people who eat the brain or spinal cord of infected animals, and it is invariably fatal. The disease sparked a public health crisis in Britain in the 1980s, and it has since appeared in the United States, Canada, western Europe, and Japan.[39] BSE arose after cattle, which naturally eat only plant material, were given remains of other ruminants in their feed as a protein supplement.[40] Since then, countries including the United States and Canada have officially banned the feeding of ruminant wastes, at least to some livestock. But completely eliminating the practice is not so easy. In 2004, a newspaper reported Canadian government statistics showing that more than half of cattle feeds tested contained animal protein materials not listed as ingredients — and they were not supposed to be there.[41] The European Union, however, is considering sanctioning the controversial practice again. Meat producers need feed sources, and South American soy comes at a high environmental cost. So the European Parliament has been debating whether to once again allow animal by-products into feed for non-ruminants such as pigs.[42]

But it is avian flus that are most worrisome for Dr. Greger, who says the most lethal of these, H5N1, has the ability to infect millions of people — and be fatal to many of them.[43] So far, there have only been a few hundred human cases of avian flu. But if that virus or a similar one should become widespread among humans, the results could be dire. The possibility for such a scenario exists, especially if animals ever became infected with a mixture of bird and swine viruses, which could combine the transmissibility of swine flu with the lethality of bird flu.[44]

Biosecurity has consequently become a buzzword in factory farming, resulting in limits on unauthorized people wandering in and out of facilities, plenty of hand-washing, and as little human-animal contact as possible. So visiting a factory farm has become almost impossible for researchers, which conveniently keeps meat production even farther from the public eye. Meanwhile, biosecurity adds another disadvantage to local farmers. Because it requires physical and technical systems and regular monitoring, it costs money that small and medium-sized livestock farms often can't rouse. Ironically, then, industrial factory farms, which bear partial responsibility for the spread of zoonoses, can more likely adhere to biosecurity requirements and be allowed to stay in business. It reminds me that technology, in this case biosecurity, sometimes advantages only the few that can afford it. But even a perceived need for biosecurity raises fundamental questions about the wisdom of the ways we make food and the impact that has on health.

Intensively Raised Livestock Get Drugs

Even if we're aware that drugs have been administered to livestock, it's sobering to hear the details. Intensively produced livestock subsist on not only grains and grasses but also quite a few pharmaceuticals. Often used as feed additives, the drugs frequently go to animals that aren't even sick.

There are lengthy lists of chemical compounds approved for livestock, as you can see on the websites of the Canadian Food Inspection

Agency (CFIA)[45] and the US Food and Drug Administration (FDA).[46] There are drugs for cattle and calves, drugs for chickens, drugs for turkeys, and drugs for swine. There are drugs for when animals get sick, or even just stressed. And there are chemicals categorized as nutritional compounds for faster weight gain, growth promotion, and feed efficiency. The drugs have long names that tempt the reader to skim. But occasionally you see one that sounds familiar (if you read it slowly), such as chlortetracycline hydrochloride — a tetracycline antibiotic. Antibiotics have sparked controversy in health care, so more on those in a moment.

Arsenic compounds are one group of feed additives that was approved and used for decades. Humorous as we may find the 1940s film comedy *Arsenic and Old Lace*, in real life, this chemical compound is a good one to avoid. Yet for years, in both the United States and Canada, intensively raised chickens and other livestock were fed a drug called 3-Nitro, or Roxarsone; its chemical name shows it to be an "arsonic" compound.[47] Statistics on use are hard to pin down, but one group of poultry scientists in the United States did the math and reported that 70% of broiler chickens got Roxarsone between 1995 and 2000.[48] The drug has for years been banned across the Atlantic, where the European Union does not agree it is benign or safe.

Happily for our health, sales of Roxarsone have recently been disallowed in both the United States and Canada. The FDA decision came after scientific investigators found that chicken livers contained the inorganic form of arsenic, which can be carcinogenic. Regulators had originally okayed Roxarsone because it contained the organic form of arsenic, which is not carcinogenic. But reports were accumulating that suggested that organic arsenic can transform into the inorganic kind in the environment. And then the arsenic started showing up in chicken livers.[49] (The idea that any form of arsenic was put into food animals had previously sparked campaigns by citizen organizations including the Center for Food Safety and Food and Water Watch.) Finally in 2011, sales of Roxarsone were ended.[50] One giant chicken maker had already said it would stop using arsenic compounds,[51] and now the pharmaceutical company that made the drug announced it would wind down sales. However, at least one further arsenic compound, nitarsone, is still approved for use in some livestock.[52]

Let's pause for a moment and muster our common sense. Why would we feed forms of arsenic to animals that we're planning to eat? Yes, these additives help produce more meat for less cost, but is that worth the possible harm? In the case just mentioned, pharmaceutical and government officials say the health risk to consumers was very low because the amount of arsenic found in the animals was very low, and the animals excreted most of the chemical.[53] But that could still unleash the drug into the environment, where it has the potential to accumulate over time.[54] Regulators had assumed that one form of arsenic wouldn't morph into a more dangerous kind. But nature is not always so predictable. This is the rationale for the precautionary principle, the international guideline suggesting caution on new practices until the evidence is in.

Another controversial livestock drug, called ractopamine, is approved in the United States and Canada for turkeys, swine, and beef to promote weight gain, feed efficiency, and lean muscle tissue.[55] Most of us have never heard of it, but one executive of an intensive meat company told me the vast majority of conventionally raised pigs receive it. Yet the drug is disallowed in China, Europe, and some other regions. So ractopamine has been a sore point between the United States and trading partners that don't want meat containing any traces of the drug.[56]

Ractopamine may be approved by our governments, but they nevertheless issue stern warnings concerning its use. According to the CFIA,[57] employees with cardiovascular disease should avoid exposure to the chemical; people who are mixing and handling the medicated feed should use protective clothing, impervious gloves, and a dust mask, and they should wash thoroughly with soap and water after handling.[58] The agency's website adds that pigs fed this drug "may be at increased risk for exhibiting the fatigued or downer pig syndrome."[59] There was an additional caution on the website — which has since been removed — stating that "turkeys fed ractopamine hydrochloride may experience alteration in behaviour, hyperexcitability, hyperactivity, musculoskeletal or cutaneous injury, and increased mortality."[60] And this drug is going into some of our meat.

When I studied undergraduate psychopharmacology at the University of Chicago, the professor said something I will never forget. "All drugs are dirty," he declared one day from the front of the classroom, riveting students with a troublesome truth. No chemical medication has ever been invented, he continued, nor would it ever, that provides solely the benefit we seek.[61] That's true whether the drug claims to promote human weight loss, improve our mood, alleviate our headaches, or make animals lean. Every drug has effects additional to those we wish, and the side effects are frequently undesirable. My professor's piece of wisdom is a reminder that there are unknowns when we mess with Mother Nature. It's one reason I avoid unnecessary medications of any kind. It's a reason for us to reconsider the chemicals we put into meat animals and agriculture as a whole. It's another argument for chemical-free food.

Hormones are an additional set of additives administered to intensively raised cattle, with the rationale that it puts more lean beef on our plates at lower prices.[62] Hormones have gotten a bad reputation, and producers who don't use them want consumers to know it. "We do not use growth hormones in the hog industry in Canada," said Mike Teillet of the Manitoba Pork Council in an informative e-mail to me.[63] Manager of Sustainable Development Programs for the council, Mr. Teillet cautions against broad criticisms and assumptions that all livestock production is the same. Pork producers, he said, are constantly improving health, environmental, and animal-welfare practices. Officials in both Canada and the United States say neither chickens nor pigs get growth hormones there.[64]

Indeed, some livestock producers are working to tone down the pharmaceuticals. In the case of beef hormones, organic and other sustainable ranchers in the United States and Canada don't use them. But most conventional beef producers do. One report estimated that two thirds of all US cattle, and as many as 90% of those on feedlots, get growth-promoting hormones.[65] Environmental advocate and cattle rancher Nicolette Hahn Niman, who opposes intensive livestock practices, also estimates that nine out of ten beef cattle in US feedlots get hormones.[66]

Hormones are often injected into animals with a special gun, which seems appropriately dramatic since these are powerful chemical messengers, responsible for regulating reproduction and other key functions in people and animals. Cattle producers and the meat industry say these pharmaceuticals are not dangerous. But it's reasonable to ask whether adding hormones to food animals is wise considering that an excess of hormones, or chemicals mimicking them, can interfere with human and animal physiology.[67] There's so much talk of the dangers of environmental hormones, that in scientific circles they're succinctly referred to as "endocrine disruptors." For non-scientists, it just doesn't seem right. While I was touring the Canadian Prairies, one of my companions, a local farmer who objects to many feedlot regimens, commented simply: "People don't realize how many hormones go into their factory-farmed beef."

The practice of giving hormones to cattle has drawn protests, including those of the American Public Health Association.[68] Citizen group Beyond Factory Farming sent a petition to the Canadian government asking for information on, and examination of, the practice. "Considering the life span of the animals, the dosages of the hormones, and the rate of excretion, the amount of hormones being released into the environment is significant," said the petition.[69] In response, the Ministry of Agriculture and AgriFood replied that testosterone from beef and other livestock is not a problem because it degrades and is neutralized in the environment. Unfortunately, such debates often just pit one group of scientific studies against another.[70]

Europe doesn't approve of hormones in beef and has banned their use. Supporting that ban is a 142-page European Commission analysis from 1999, stating that hormones in meat can impair immune and nervous systems.[71] European countries won't buy hormone-treated North American meat, a decision that has caused a long-running dispute between the two continents. On the American side, governments and producers argue not so much over the health data as over whether free trade agreements allow Europe to exclude North American meat.[72]

This suggests to me that economic considerations too often trump health concerns.

Health officials have wondered for years whether beef hormones might be contributing to the disturbing trend toward early puberty in children.[73] While I was conducting research, a front-page story in a Canadian national newspaper announced recent findings on the phenomenon.[74] Girls in New York, Cincinnati, and San Francisco had been found to be developing breasts and pubic hair as early as seven years old, especially girls who were obese.[75]

Young-onset puberty has been documented for decades, and analysts have suggested factors including too many calories, too many fatty foods, and exposure to endocrine-disrupting chemicals.[76] There's no evidence of a role for beef hormones specifically, but chemicals approved for cattle do include estradiol, progesterone, and testosterone, the hormones that regulate human reproduction.[77]

Meanwhile, research has suggested that heavy meat consumption — even without extra hormones — might be linked to earlier onset of menstrual periods in young girls.[78] Dr. Imogen Rogers and colleagues in the UK published a rigorous study in 2010[79] involving more than 3,000 girls. They discovered that the girls who had consumed more than twelve portions of meat a week at age seven were more likely to have started their menstrual periods by age 12½ than were girls who had eaten less meat. I communicated with the lead author, who confirmed that the children in the study were born after the 1980s, when hormone-treated meat was banned in Europe. Large amounts of animal protein itself appear to contribute to the trend, she said.[80]

There is no single answer to what is causing early puberty. Kids grow up quickly these days for a lot of reasons, including increased access to media and sex-related images, and economic and cultural shifts that have lessened the control parents traditionally had over children and teens. Then there are further biological factors such as non-food environmental chemicals.[81] Whatever the factors, early puberty is worrisome. It's a signal for the start of sexual activity, potential pregnancy, and adult responsibilities for which children are rarely prepared.

How much meat we eat, and the ways we allow it to be produced, are all intertwined. It's a lot to chew on as we consider what kinds of food systems we want for our communities and our health.

Antibiotics Are in a Class of Their Own

Of all our pharmaceuticals today, one group's overuse has caused a full-on public health crisis: antibiotics. They're the wonder drugs that transformed 20th-century medicine by combating bacterial infections. But antibiotics are now so environmentally pervasive that bacteria are learning to cope, and the world is experiencing the rise of antibiotic-resistant bacteria against which humans have no medicinal defense. The problem hit the news when immune "superbugs" starting spreading through communities and even medical clinics. Superbugs are typified by the multidrug-resistant *Staphylococcus aureus* (MRSA), which kills thousands of Americans a year.[82] Health officials have significantly lowered the number of hospital-initiated MRSA infections, but it remains a serious public health concern.[83]

For the proliferation of antibiotics, the medical community has been assumed to be the culprit. It's true that medical antibiotics have at times been liberally employed, although patients deserve some blame for expecting chemical solutions to every ache and pain. A physician friend of mine tells me some patients get angry if she refuses to prescribe antibiotics, even if what they have is the common cold — a viral infection that won't respond to those drugs.

But livestock and meat production represent the really profligate use of antibiotics. Recent FDA data suggest that 70% or more of the antibiotics used in the United States go to livestock.[84] The drugs can make animals grow bigger faster, as well as lessening animal illness in the indoor conditions of CAFOs. At least one massive pork producer in the United States has been working to cut back,[85] and in Europe, antibiotics in food animals have declined considerably since 2006, when the European Union banned the drugs when used purely for growth promotion. Yet even in Europe, the World Health Organization comments that too many antibiotics are still being used, which could compromise human health.[86] The FDA defends the use of antibiotics if the drugs are employed judiciously.[87]

The widespread use of these chemicals means it's no coincidence that the antibiotic-resistant bacteria MRSA has been found in livestock and meat. One Midwestern hog factory showed high levels of MRSA in both the hogs and the people working there.[88] A study in 2012 found MRSA in almost 7% of retail pork samples from stores in Iowa, Minnesota, and New Jersey.[89]

Public health expert Dr. Ellen Silbergeld co-authored a powerful review of the problem of antibiotic resistance.[90] She's professor and editor-in-chief for Environmental Research at Johns Hopkins Bloomberg School of Public Health, and has a long list of achievements, including being named a MacArthur Foundation "Genius" Fellow and receiving Fulbright and other fellowships. She has been scientific advisor to the EPA, the World Bank, the UN Environmental Program, the Centers for Disease Control, and other organizations.[91] Dr. Silbergeld considers antibiotic resistance a major public health problem, and she points the finger squarely at meat production.

There are four lines of evidence implicating intensive livestock practices in antibiotic resistance, says Dr. Silbergeld. First, making meat accounts for a major use of antibiotics worldwide. Second, many antibiotics for livestock are given subtherapeutically to animals that are not ill — a tactic especially likely to produce resistance. Third, meat production uses antibiotics of key clinical types, including those used for humans. Fourth, as a result of all these factors, human populations are now regularly exposed to antibiotic-resistant disease agents in their environments. Dr. Silbergeld may be a cautious academic, but she candidly describes some factory farms as "comparable to poorly run hospitals" where virtually everyone gets antibiotics, patients lie in unchanged beds, and hygiene is questionable.[92]

Other researchers agree that the problem is magnified by intensive meat facilities, where scientists have found antibiotic-resistant bacteria in livestock, other animals, and employees. Insects around factory farms can pick up antibiotic-resistant bacteria from swine, then carry the bacteria into the environment.[93] Administering antibiotics to chickens can cause resistance, but when producers stop using a drug, resistance to it can decrease significantly, as has been shown in Quebec chicken hatcheries.[94] So, the problem is solvable, if we just stop overusing these drugs. When new antibiotics are introduced to livestock, researchers find more resistant bacteria in humans nearby. For example, resistance to the antibiotic fluoroquinolone spiked to 80% in humans shortly after its introduction to the livestock industry in Spain, but human resistance to this drug is low in Australia, where it has never been used in agriculture.[95] Other jurisdictions have witnessed a decline in the problem after bans on livestock antibiotics.

Here's how subtherapeutic administration causes resistance: Where high doses of antibiotics would kill all the bacteria in the pigs and cattle, low doses diminish the microbes but don't overwhelm them. Some continue living and reproducing, especially those with random genetic resistance to the drug. Over time, immune bacteria come to dominate. In this way, subtherapeutic use of antibiotics selects for more and more resistant bacteria. Finally, a point is reached where the bacteria are unperturbed by the antimicrobial agent and are happily in a state of resistance.

You'd think they'd use different antibiotics in cattle, chickens, and pigs than they use in people, if only to minimize the development of resistance in important human medicines. But some antibiotics for livestock are similar to those used for people, including tetracyclines, penicillins, and sulfa drugs.[96] That's one reason "almost every type of clinically relevant bacteria has developed antibiotic resistance," as the Centers for Disease Control official Dr. Ali Khan testified to the US government in 2010.[97]

"Poultry Industry Warned to Halt Use of Antibiotic," said the front-page headline in a local newspaper.[98] Grocery-store chicken had been tested by Canada's public health agency, which had found increased levels of drug-resistant *Campylobacter*, a food-borne bug that can make people sick. So the agency is warning meat producers to moderate their use of antibiotics. It's part of a growing wave of calls for cutbacks to livestock drugs. The issue is bound to be a heated one, since some intensive producers consider antibiotics essential to raising large numbers of animals in close quarters. We can help antibiotics stay essential to human health by scaling back on our intake of animal products, purchasing ones that are chemical-free, and reminding ourselves about the importance of antibiotics that work.

Lifestyle Diseases Get a Hand from Too Much Meat

When I first started studying health and disease, I was fascinated by the macabre topic of what is killing people today. Turn back the clock a century, and you'll find the major causes of death were infectious diseases such as pneumonia and flus.[99] The current epidemiological landscape is very different. You may know of individuals who died tragically of infectious diseases, or AIDS, or accidents, and these loom large in our memories. But the most common causes of death in high-income countries are cardiovascular diseases (including heart conditions and stroke) and cancers. Those two categories account for more than 50% of all deaths in the United States[100] and close to 40% of all deaths in high-income countries.[101] People still die of infections, especially in developing countries. But the biggest individual killers in the world, and increasingly even in poor nations, are heart conditions, stroke, and cancer.

These medical problems are now commonly referred to as "lifestyle diseases." But I continue to be struck by the profound nature of the phenomenon. Heart disease, stroke, and cancer are linked to so-called lifestyle diseases because they are heavily influenced by our choices. Which means we have agency. If we choose to exercise it, we have power. That does not mean it's your fault if you suffer from any such syndromes. Heart disease, cancers, and other chronic ailments are complex and multifactorial, so any particular individual may have heart problems or cancer for reasons of genetic predisposition or other factors over which they have no control. But as a whole, lifestyle syndromes get that label because they can be influenced by our choices.

To lower our vulnerability to heart disease, cancers, and other chronic ailments, it helps if we don't smoke, keep our stress in check, and get regular exercise. It also helps to watch our food choices,[102] and going easy on animal products is part of the prescription. Studies show that partial or full vegetarians are less prone to chronic disease — and tend to be healthier overall — than heavy meat-eaters. It's true that people we could call meat minimizers are more likely to eat good fibrous foods, not smoke, and otherwise take care of themselves, but scientists have teased out those variables and shown that, for most of us, less meat leads to more health.[103]

To explain chronic disease, it helps to recognize the role of simple overeating.[104] Many of us regularly consume to excess these days, as our ancient brains respond to an abundance of heavily advertised, relatively cheap processed foods. Fatty, salty, and sugary snacks are everywhere. So we reach for these, which get produced en masse at economies of scale, driving the price down and encouraging us to buy more. As much as 40% of the increased prevalence in obesity in the past 25 years may be attributable to the reduced unit price of processed foods.[105] It's a major reason that today, though close to a billion individuals on the planet are undernourished or starving, more than a billion are overweight or obese.[106] According to one analysis, average Americans each consume 1,000 excess calories a day, roughly 30–40% more than they need.[107] We're encouraged by hefty portion sizes at restaurants, a symbol for consumption overall.

Even in developing countries, for which the stereotype is that people are thin, many citizens have overburdened bodies and related health problems, while others are tragically undernourished.[108] Statisticians call this situation a "bimodal distribution," which means that two different trends exist at the same time. A sobering two thirds of adult Americans are either overweight or obese,[109] and that percentage is expected to rise to a shocking 75% by 2020.[110] A full one third, or 34.4%, of Americans qualify as obese, as do 24.1% of Canadians.[111] One half of Americans have a health problem for which they take a prescription drug each week.[112] Some people regularly choose hamburgers, fries, and ice cream, then pop pills to lower their cholesterol. In some sense today, to be fat and unhealthy is to be normal.

A century ago, many of our ancestors genuinely worried whether they would get enough sustenance, and officials encouraged people to eat heartily. But today's problem is often the opposite, and it is not government but producers who encourage us to indulge. Too many calories, especially the wrong kind, now kill as many people as smoking does, according to acclaimed nutrition professor and author Marion Nestle. Food and cigarettes each contribute to about one fifth of annual US deaths.[113]

Exercise is also a factor in obesity and related health problems. Food corporations would like us to believe it's the main factor, and they've spent public relations money on playgrounds and school exercise programs.[114] But eating habits deserve much of the blame.[115] Meat is not the whole problem, but it's a key component of the Standard American Diet, which is SAD, indeed, in the view of food writer Mark Bittman, an articulate advocate for lower-meat diets.[116]

An overabundance of animal-source foods loads us with cholesterol and fat, which can contribute to cardiovascular disease, hypertension, stroke, Type II diabetes, and other problems.[117] The evidence is strong enough that even scientific articles state the problem unequivocally: "The high level of meat and saturated fat consumption in the USA and other high-income countries exceeds nutritional needs and contributes to high rates of chronic diseases," say public health experts at Johns Hopkins University.[118]

Heart disease and stroke, often grouped together as cardiovascular disease, account for almost one third of all deaths in the United States.[119] Cardiovascular disease is encouraged by animal-heavy diets, so people who consume large amounts of meat, dairy products, and eggs are more vulnerable.[120] When we base our diets mostly on meat and dairy, we get regular servings of saturated fats and cholesterol, which can increase blood cholesterol levels and raise our risk of heart problems.[121] Nutrition scientists argue about the details, such as the degree to which dietary cholesterol raises blood cholesterol and the role of factors such as genetics and other life choices. Additionally, they point out that non-meat sources such as trans-fatty acids can also raise blood cholesterol. But the fact remains that people who eat less meat tend to have less chance of developing heart problems.

Of all the years lost to heart disease, many could be saved if people just lowered their meat intake to environmentally sustainable levels, according to one study. If the UK and Brazil adhered to international gas emissions targets and lowered meat production and consumption by

30% by 2030, it would save at least 15% of the years that would have been lost to heart disease.[122]

Stroke is the term used to describe brain conditions in which blood vessels burst or are blocked, interfering with the normal flow of blood and oxygen we need for cognition, physical movement, and general functioning. Risk factors include smoking, plentiful alcohol consumption, minimal physical activity, and high blood pressure.[123] Though meat consumption isn't considered a particular risk factor for stroke, this devastating disease is more likely in people who eat badly and often. You're more likely to suffer stroke if you have poor heart health and diabetes, which can be fueled by excessive intake of animal products.

Cancer is also high on the list of diseases exacerbated by too much meat. Most of the research has implicated red and processed varieties, but too much of other meats may also raise your risk. Cancer has many contributing factors, including bad luck either in genetics or environment. Yet a consistent finding has been that heavy meat-eaters are more vulnerable than people who eat little or none.

The main objects of study have been red meats and processed types, like hot dogs and salamis, that have been cured, salted, and gussied up.[124] One group of researchers at the National Institutes of Health in Bethesda, Maryland, has conducted numerous studies linking meat consumption to cancer. Using data from half a million Americans, they showed that high consumers of red and processed meats were more likely to get cancers of various kinds. The more red meat people ate, the more likely they were to develop cancers including esophageal, colorectal, and liver. The more processed meat people ate, the more likely they were to get colorectal and lung cancers.[125] Other research also shows that daily meat-eaters appear to have greater risk of colon cancer than do people who rarely eat meat.[126] One meta-analysis of numerous studies showed a relationship between stomach cancer and heavy consumption of processed meats like bacon.[127] Too much meat of any kind can play a role in cancer, and one study showed that "women, both pre- and post-menopausal, who consumed the most meat had the highest risk of breast cancer."[128] Investigations by the World Cancer Research Fund and the American Institute for Cancer Research have shown for years that people who limit their meat intake are less likely to develop cancer.[129] As those expert bodies recommend on their website, "eat mostly foods of plant origin."[130]

Factory-farmed meat gives us not only saturated fat and cholesterol, but also the proliferation of chemicals in our environment. Pesticides and fertilizers, widely used in livestock feed, can disrupt immune systems and cause various pathologies.[131] And while pesticide use for feed production has declined in some regions (in the amount applied per unit of land), many pesticides are now more toxic than before.[132]

Diabetes is also on the rise and is now a fact of life for tens of millions of Americans. According to the US Centers for Disease Control, more than 8% of Americans have it, but if you also count those with pre-diabetes, you're talking about one third of the national population.[133] Diabetics are susceptible to kidney failure, blindness, heart disease, and other serious conditions.[134] Genetic predisposition plays a role, but it's a medical reality that many Type II diabetics are overweight and eat high-calorie diets. Type II is the diabetes most diagnosed today, and studies show you're more vulnerable if you're a heavy consumer of red and processed meats.[135] Television chef Paula Deen, famous for meaty southern meals and recipes including her "Lady's Brunch Burger" (ground beef, bacon, butter, and eggs, with a liberal dose of salty seasoning, optionally stacked between glazed donuts) revealed late in 2011 that she has Type II diabetes.[136] Ms. Deen has since made an arrangement with a pharmaceutical company to promote a diabetes drug. She has also said her recipes will lighten up.[137]

Anchoring the research on food and health is the authoritative book *The China Study*.[138] It was co-authored by T. Colin Campbell, professor of nutritional biochemistry at Cornell University, who oversaw a comprehensive 20-year study on links between diet and health in China and Taiwan. Finding more than 8,000 statistically significant associations between what we eat and the diseases we get, the study suggested that people who eat the most animal-based foods tend to get the most chronic disease, and that those who eat the most plant-based foods tend to be healthiest, with the least chronic disease.[139] It showed that people are more likely to get cancer if they consume large amounts of animal protein, and that the danger is not just from additives, but from excessive amounts of meat itself. The study also found evidence that chronic disease is not inevitable based on genetics. Genes don't have effects until they are triggered or "expressed" by conditions in the person's body or environment, and that can include food. Though residents of China have a high degree of genetic similarity, in some regions they suffer much more cancer than in others, and it tends to be where residents eat more meat.[140]

Healthy Solutions Include Eating Less and Better

Most of us grew up hearing that meat and milk would build strong bones, that we needed large amounts of protein, and that the more we ate, especially from animals, the healthier we'd be. But science is documenting that you can, indeed, get too much of a good thing.

After years of avoiding this topic, some health agencies are pointing to meat and suggesting, explicitly or implicitly, that we respond. The British Columbia Cancer Agency says that for colorectal cancer, "risk increases with higher dietary fat and meat consumption, and lower fiber, fruit and vegetable consumption."[141] Emphasizing the positive, one high-profile 2007 study noted that we have an opportunity "to prevent cancer and improve global health" if we "limit intake of red meat and avoid processed meat."[142] That study, from the American Institute for Cancer Research and the World Cancer Research Fund, also said that to help avoid cancer, one important overall step is to eat less meat.

There are also solutions available to solve the antibiotics problem. Many agencies are working to end the overuse of antibiotics in meat production. The US Centers for Disease Control, the World Health Organization, the UN Food and Agriculture Organization, the Pew Commission on Industrial Farm Animal Production, and a growing list of additional groups have called for restrictions on antimicrobials in livestock production. Numerous European countries have taken action. And there is a taste in the corridors of Washington to limit antibiotics for livestock growth promotion. Meanwhile, consumers can make the commitment to move away from conventionally produced meat.

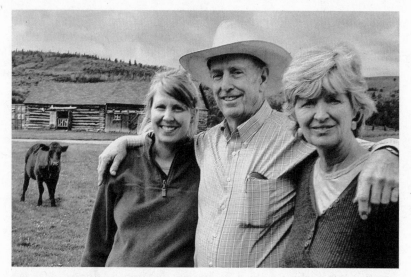

"We turn cellulose into beef." Francis Gardner (center) with his wife Bonnie (R) and daughter Sarah (L) on their Mount Sentinel Ranch in southern Alberta, where they produce organic sustainable beef.

All such steps toward healthier meat rouse opposition from some people in agribusiness who argue that such shifts will increase prices. They're right that healthier meat production will probably raise retail prices for animal products. As consumers and part of society, we will be presented with what could be a tough choice. Do we want inexpensive bacon and wings if they come at the cost of our health? Or do we want to pay more for robust environments and well-being?

To take the healthy high road, we can support producers like Francis Gardner and his family, who produce organic beef at Mount Sentinel Ranch in the rolling southern Alberta countryside. I had the opportunity to visit the Gardners when I drove to their ranch in the mountain foothills southwest of Calgary. There I met Francis, his wife Bonnie and daughter Sarah, along with neighbor Gordon Cartwright, who dropped over to share their ideas about producing livestock in ways that support rather than degrade the environment.

These ranchers use no antibiotics or hormones on their animals, and no chemical fertilizers or herbicides on the land. What they do at Mount Sentinel Ranch is what traditional cattle ranchers do. "We convert cellulose into beef," observes Mr. Gardner. Cattle at Mount Sentinel graze for about a year and a half, muscling up to 900–950 pounds. At that point, they are either slaughtered or fattened a little more in natural feedlots. The organic beef is sold under the label Diamond Willow.

The Gardners graze their few hundred cattle on native rangeland, including on the legendary groundcover "rough fescue," which inspires a kind of reverence. It's a mix of dozens of species, hardy and diverse, with deep roots and tolerance for extreme and varied weather conditions, and it sustained buffalo and other livestock for thousands of years. There's still rough fescue on the higher hills and some of the ranges that local residents are trying to steward.

Stewardship is the point for the Gardners. This ranch has been operating since 1898, when the property was purchased by Francis Gardner's grandfather. Today, the ranch reminds them of past generations, and it makes them think about future ones. That's why it's certified organic, and that's why they only graze the number of cattle that can be supported by the grassy groundcover. "You're trying to minimize your impact on the land," says Mr. Gardner. Producers like the Gardners receive a premium for their beef. But the main reason they produce organically is knowing that they're doing the right thing for the land, for communities, and for the well-being of customers. They're holding out for a different way of making beef and for a food system that adds to local control, environmental sustainability, and human health.

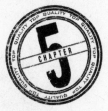

Food Systems Should Reflect Our Values

We Want Quality of Life

Elsie Herring used to sit outside on her rural North Carolina property, chatting with others and breathing the country air. It was a satisfying part of life on land that had been in her family since they came out of slavery. She and her mother and brother lived there, along with other family, on a dead-end road near a place called Rockfish Creek. Now there's just Ms. Herring left, and friendly neighbors.

But there's no more sitting outside. Since a factory farm went in nearby years ago, Ms. Herring has been subjected to hog waste blowing on her house, her property, and herself. Like other citizens in the rural United States, Canada, and around the world whose lives were changed after CAFOs moved in, she spends a lot of time indoors. "It's like living in prison in your own house," she told me when I visited North Carolina. "That odor is something," she said. "You can smell it all the time. You can't open your windows. There are more flies and other insects. You can't go outside." The water is dirty, and one of Ms. Herring's neighbors who got hers tested was told by water-quality officials: "Don't drink the water. Don't cook in it. Don't let the dog drink it." There's no hanging laundry on the line, unless you want the clothing spotted with manure. The residents buy bottled water and take their clothing to the laundromat, she said. "Our basic human rights are being violated."[1]

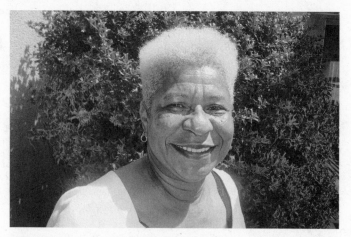

"That odor is something." Elsie Herring, rural resident of North Carolina, has been experiencing livestock pollution first-hand since an intensive hog operation moved into her neighborhood.

It's no coincidence that Ms. Herring is African American. As demonstrated in a detailed geographical analysis by epidemiologist Dr. Steve Wing and his colleagues at the University of North Carolina, CAFOs are especially prevalent in areas that are both poor and black.[2] Especially when meat factories are run by the largest and most powerful producers, they are five times as likely to be located in regions that have a high percentage of non-whites. The academic article called it "environmental injustice," but it's "environmental racism" to Naeema Muhammed, a community organizer with the North Carolina Environmental Justice Network.[3] In an interview, she suggested low-income African American communities are "avenues of least resistance." For CAFOs, those regions are where land is cheapest. But that's also where there's the least likelihood of protest.

Pig factories do not go into wealthy neighborhoods. In 1997, a pork producer proposed to locate in Moore County, south of the state capital of Raleigh, which would have placed hog barns in an affluent community near a posh golf course. The proposal never went through.[4] Activists would like to see ordinary neighborhoods have that kind of clout, so they advise local residents of their rights and encourage them to challenge the factory farms.

Meeting Ms. Herring was one of those research experiences that brought the scientific studies off the page for me. It reminded me that CAFO problems are not just lists of statistics. The real-life facts are that livestock produce large amounts of waste, and that thousands of animals crowded into small buildings produce so much of it that it infringes on the lives of nearby residents. The problem has been documented by Dr. Kendall Thu, an anthropology professor at Northern Illinois University. He has observed the impact of industrial livestock production, and says:

> "Ask neighbors of an industrial hog operation in rural Saskatchewan or North Carolina about their experiences. In vivid detail they will describe their diminished quality of life, the impairment of surface and groundwater, the horrific odor, the social upheaval and divisions among neighbors, friends, and family members, the displacement of family farmers and rural decay, the inequitable burden placed on impoverished rural neighborhoods and communities of color, concerns over health problems from airborne emissions, intimidation by local officials and industry representatives, and the collusion between industry, government, and research institutions."[5]

Other researchers have demonstrated reduced quality of life by measuring factors such as the number of times residents can or cannot open their windows or spend time outdoors. Living near a factory farm can increase tension, depression, anger, fatigue, and physical ailments.[6]

For Ms. Herring, even if she wanted to move from her ancestral home to escape the pollution and discomfort, she'd have trouble getting a decent price because not many people want to buy land next to a factory farm.[7] Economics professor William Weida has written widely about this and related issues and is president of the Idaho-based Socially Responsible Agriculture Project. Dr. Weida has demonstrated that property values frequently drop when a factory farm comes to the neighborhood. Communities become undesirable and people move away, fueling a depopulation that has devastating consequences for the countryside.[8]

Conflict is another sign of the diminishing quality of rural life. When an agribusiness company applies to set up an intensive livestock operation, confusion and social tension arise as local residents argue how to handle this tidal wave of change. Applications by factory farms can result in protests, picketing, and contentious community meetings where tempers flare. A proposal in 1993 for a 4,000-sow intensive livestock operation (ILO) in Manitoba sparked such local opposition that police were called in to one meeting to restore order, as documented by Winnipeg sociologist Dr. Joel Novek.[9] Construction on the facility eventually began, but one day "the partially completed structure mysteriously burned to the ground."[10] The factories can drive a wedge between neighbors and within families. Some people argue that ILOs or CAFOs are good for the community — or at least inevitable — and others are determined to fight. Brothers argue, and friends stop speaking.

The conflicts that accompany establishment of new ILOs have contributed to a subtle but widespread change in rural life. Farm communities used to be relatively cohesive, with people linked by shared expectations about stewarding the land. Neighbors helped each other and socialized together. Today, rural communities have less of what researchers call "social capital" — mutual trust and reliance, reciprocity, and shared identity and norms.[11]

I don't romanticize farming. It's hard work, and it's not for all of us. Personally, I don't have the considerable skills needed. But farm life appeals to some people. It's outdoor work focused on the basics of life. It requires independence and self-reliance, and it allows families to engage in the earthy, but meaningful, work of providing sustenance for themselves and others. Those who long for that life should be able to have it — and earn a good living and respect as providers of our basic needs. But opportunities have decreased for individuals and families to farm. Ironically, the "right to farm" (RTF) now applies largely to corporations. Most or all jurisdictions in Canada and the United States have some form of RTF laws, which can end up shielding industrial farming from citizen complaints about everything from odor and pollution to control of agricultural markets.[12] We need to give the right to farm back to those who provide quality food and add to our quality of life.

We Want Local Control

It used to be, you could drive through rural areas and see a diverse mix of small and medium-sized acreages, the countryside dotted with grazing cows and farmhouses. Today, in many regions, you're more likely to see expanses of single crops or long windowless buildings that are invisibly packed with livestock. Not many people or animals in sight. Not many smallholdings with a variety of crops, or animals foraging, or people doing farm chores. Not much of what is generally referred to as the family farm.

The "decline of the family farm" is a phrase that has been used so much that it has lost its power to shock. Yet it describes a cultural upheaval that has occurred largely without public awareness or discussion. For decades, there has been exodus from rural agricultural areas as farmers and their children leave the land, voluntarily or not, and take up city life. In the United States and Canada, the number of agricultural operations has been declining for a century, while the size of the remaining farms has expanded. Many small farmers live in poverty. If they go bankrupt, the land often gets further consolidated in the hands of a few. Traditional rural life has faded in what farmer-writer Thomas Pawlick has termed a "great dying."[13]

In 1900, about 40% of Americans lived and worked on farms. Today it is 2%.[14] The numbers are about the same for Canada, where in 1931 (when the counting began) almost one in every three Canadians lived on farms, but by 2006, it was close to one in 50.[15] Farm closures have been occurring for decades, but in the past 20 years alone the number of farms in Canada has declined by more than one quarter, to 215,000 today.[16] The data are less extreme globally, but show the same trend.[17] Dairy farms provide a dramatic example. In the United States, 95% of dairy operations disappeared in the past half century; there were more than 3.5 million farms in 1950, but only 65,000 in 2009.[18] Most were replaced by high-technology facilities churning out milk products en masse. Mega-dairies have come to dominate the industry, especially in the western states.[19] Meanwhile, in the United States, for all types of livestock, in just the five years between 2002 and 2007, the number of factory-farmed animals increased significantly.[20]

One of the impediments to vibrant local farming communities is corporate concentration of agriculture. In the United States, four companies control more than 80% of the beef industry, making it more centralized and concentrated than it was in the early 20th century, when writer Upton Sinclair wrote his meat factory exposé *The Jungle*. [21] Most of the market for pork is similarly controlled by a small number of companies.[22] Just 2% of livestock facilities raise 40% of all animals.[23] The trend is to aggregation, and many small farmers have gone broke. It's different in Canadian chicken production, which is "supply managed" so independent producers can compete. But even in Canada, the food system is highly oligopolistic, much of it controlled by just a few large corporations.[24]

Multinational agribusinesses gain their influence partly by owning every level of an industry from start to finish. In some cases, they breed the animals, fatten them, slaughter them, and then sell their meat at retail. That's why they're called "vertically integrated," or "integrators." According to one pork company, it has control "from squeal to meal."[25] Increasingly, animals are raised under contracts between integrators and farmers who are called "contract growers." Growers run day-to-day operations, while the integrator owns the animals and sets policies on matters from livestock feed to farm infrastructure.[26] Agricultural writers have criticized the system as giving too much power to integrators and too much financial risk to growers.[27] Only 11% of hogs in the United States were sold under such agreements in 1993, but by 2004, that percentage had jumped to 69%.[28]

It's tempting to shrug at these trends and call them progress. Many of us imagine that small farms must not be productive enough to feed a hungry world. Yet recent research suggests that small farms can be efficient producers while operating more sustainably than large and intensive ones. They can, in some cases, yield more food per unit of land while requiring less energy, draining less fresh water, and leaving less pollution.[29]

This notion sounds counterintuitive in a technological time when most of us believe bigger means better, and repeat the mantra of economies of scale. Yet research has shown that larger farms tend to be more efficient mostly by one narrow measure — how much of a single crop the land will yield per acre. Small farms are more likely to be engaged in polyculture rather than monoculture. They're more likely to be growing a mix of species "utilizing different root depths, plant heights, or nutrients on the same piece of land simultaneously."[30] So a giant acreage can produce more bushels of soybeans per unit area than can a small farm. But when you count total food, of all types, produced per unit of land, smaller farms are sometimes most efficient. Agricultural systems expert Peter Rosset wrote a detailed report to "challenge the conventional wisdom that small farms are backward and unproductive."[31] In it, he demonstrated the multifunctionality of small acreages and showed that some can bring forth many times as much food as industrial agribusiness, while using fewer resource inputs.[32] Agroecologist Miguel Altieri has also argued that moderate-scale farming can be highly productive using minimal land and water, and it can be resilient in the face of climate change.[33] Modest-sized farms are also more likely to create only as much waste as can be integrated into ecosystems. The United Nations agrees on the value of small-scale agriculture, and in a recent World Economic and Social Survey, the UN called for a focus on independent local farmers to feed a growing population.[34] The FAO has published "Save and Grow," a guide to supporting smallholder production, and intensifying it in ways that are sustainable, to satisfy the world's long-term food needs.[35]

Today however, even when small and independent farms are well managed, they sometimes have trouble surviving. They don't have the same encouragement from public policy, as we'll see in Chapter 8. Government programs tend to directly or indirectly assist big operations by lowering their input costs, helping with waste management, assisting with international trade, and many other measures. Small farms don't usually have the same access to distribution and marketing networks, and they don't have the capital to compete against technology-based operations run by large farm companies. In this environment, financial struggles are not necessarily signs of inefficiency.

There's something wrong with an agricultural system that has trouble accommodating independent farms, especially ones that can respond to local needs and produce more food with less environmental damage. Local farms have local allegiances that industrialized farms do not. Local farmers tend to hire local people and spend their money in the community. They often purchase inputs, such as seed, fertilizers, feeds, and animals, from nearby sellers. In contrast, industrialized operations often make decisions at the head office, purchase inputs from afar, import employees, and don't leave profits in the community.

In her corner of agricultural North America, organic farmer Colleen Ross has seen the change. Where she and her family raise crops and livestock not far from Ottawa, Ontario, the land used to be dotted with small dairies and mixed agricultural holdings owned and managed by people whose ancestors had established there. Today, most farms have either been taken over by large agricultural corporations or are growing single crops from genetically modified seeds they've purchased under contract to agribusiness. Ms. Ross has witnessed first-hand the demise of the agricultural model that formed the basis of food production for thousands of years — and its replacement by mega-farms and factories. Particularly concerned about the power of biotechnology companies, Ms. Ross has spoken about the issue at international meetings and in local town halls as a representative of the National Farmers' Union.

I had wanted to visit Ms. Ross and had the chance one autumn, when she was cleaning up the farm after harvest before winter set in. The weather was cool and the ground muddy, so Colleen loaned me some sturdy gumboots so we could have a look around. Cows and sheep trotted in and out of the open barns, and chickens pecked around the grounds. In the packing shed, there were piles of homegrown hay for the livestock, and boxes of green and red peppers left over from the last week's farmers' market.

One of the region's few independent organic operations, this farm shouldn't really exist by federal agriculture standards. The farm is too small and doesn't fit the industrialized norm. But it's an example of how much food can be coaxed from small, well-run acreages. Ms. Ross and her family grow tomatoes, peppers, and other vegetables, grains such as rye, and pulses such as soybeans, along with naturally raised beef, chicken, and lamb.[36] Their 200 acres yield annual harvests of tens of tons of soybeans; tons of grains; 40 different species of vegetables (2–8 varieties of each); and 8–10 different types of tomatoes. The operation sustains not only Colleen's family but many others, employs up to nine people, and adds to the health of the land and the people who eat what they produce. It's all done without pesticides, antibiotics, synthetic fertilizers, or genetic engineering. The harvest is the product of a healthy farm environment and the family's years of expertise.

By some measures, there still exist large numbers of family farms, but the numbers depend on how you define "family farm." Some agribusiness executives refer to themselves in public (and to the government) as family farmers, though they raise tens of thousands of animals in factories. And some family farmers stay in business by working with (or for) integrators on various aspects of livestock production; in the process, they give up considerable control of what often used to be their own operation.[37] Contract growing is not the same as independent farming. In the view of Missouri-based agricultural economist John Ikerd: "It is a factory job that just happens to involve animals."[38]

A new kind of colonization is what Dr. Ikerd calls industrial agriculture. In his essay, "Corporate Livestock Production: Implications for Rural North America," Dr. Ikerd describes parallels with political colonization that are chilling.[39] Historical takeovers of territory carried out by nations such as Britain and France are not so different from today's takeovers by corporations. A livestock company comes into a rural area proposing an intensive operation. Local people are made to feel backward, even primitive, and incapable of managing their own affairs. They're promised jobs, incomes, and shiny urban-style lives. Local economies are then slowly overpowered by the outsiders, who have little commitment to the colonies except as vehicles of wealth creation for themselves, according to Dr. Ikerd. Ultimately, rural residents find their livelihoods and communities undermined.[40]

Local control is diminished when factory farming takes over. Small-scale livestock producers can find themselves squeezed out of markets and unable to continue working on farms that may have been in the family for generations. Because meat multinationals control the sector from start to finish, they supply their processing plants with animals from their own factory farms. Pretty soon, independent producers have few places to sell. Half of Canadian hog farmers abandoned the business between 1991 and 2001.[41] While some voluntarily chose a different life, others could be said to have been pushed out.[42] Meanwhile, the number of pigs per farm has multiplied considerably. Most surviving livestock farms have had to get big.

"My wife grew up in a small mixed farm in the 1950s and 1960s, and they were poor. My father-in-law didn't want any of his kids to take over the farm. He wanted them to go out and get a 'real job' where they could earn a good living. I heard him say it many times." It's a chilling narrative, told to me by an executive in intensive livestock. The story would ring true for many families, echoing the pain of poverty and the new agricultural reality that encouraged them to abandon the farm. In one sense, such choices were voluntary, but in another sense, they were not.

Rural jobs have undergone radical changes under industrial agriculture. If you're working in meat production today, there's a chance you're in a corporate slaughterhouse. You're glad to have employment, but not so glad to be spending a shift grabbing chickens and hanging them upside down on conveyor belts. As documented by Eric Schlosser in *Fast Food Nation*, employees in processing plants are required to kill animals at high speed and work with sharp knives and machinery while hurried and stressed.[43] If you work for one of these companies, you might hold one of the limited number of jobs working directly with animals, but what you do is quite different from what your parents or grandparents did. Your father or grandmother may have worked their own places, and had 10 or 100 animals alongside a mix of crops. They would have owned and managed the farm, applying their knowledge and judgment for the good of the business and the family. Fast forward 50 years, the ancestral farm is boarded up, and you're working in a system in which control is not in your local region but in boardrooms far away.

For individuals and for communities, this is all part of massive economic and social shifts that have occurred in the countryside. Anthropologist Kendall Thu sums up the critical view: "It is simply better for the social and economic fabric of rural communities to have more farmers producing food than to have production concentrated in the hands of a few."[44]

The idea that society needs local farms isn't just nostalgia. We don't need these farms just so city-dwellers can take a drive on weekends to enjoy the sight of grazing cattle and big red barns. Family farms have been the basis of rural stability and food production for hundreds of years, and they are needed for the health of our communities. There are sweeping social and psychological consequences to loss of control. Individuals and communities need to feel they have influence over their lives. When groups of people lack such influence, they lack satisfaction and security — in this case, in terms of both livelihood and food. We can reverse this trend and take back our food systems by supporting livestock production that is sustainable, compassionate, and locally controlled.

We Want Food Systems to Strengthen Environmental Health

It's difficult to believe that too many livestock and too much meat could be the cause of so much grief. But as we have seen in the first half of this book, it is. Excessive industrial meat production causes a list of problems for the environment, for human physical and mental well-being, and for community.[45] It uses too much land and water and creates too much in the way of gas emissions and pollution. Intensive production encourages consumers — especially consumers in wealthy countries — to take more than is good for the planet or themselves.

It's all related to health, which is broadly defined by the World Health Organization as overall physical, mental, and social well-being. Or we could think of it as environmental health, encompassing both short-term and long-term well-being for ourselves, for the natural world, and for the other people and species with whom we share the earth.

Biodiversity — or rather, the loss of it — is an example of the breadth and depth of the consequences of too much meat. Essential to environmental health, biodiversity is a measure of the variety and number of plant and animal species on the planet. Roughly, the more we have the better, as in the American folk song: "All God's Creatures Got a Place in the Choir."[46] Given the complexity of ecosystems, and the number of interconnected types of plants and animals, killing off species always has negative consequences beyond those we might predict. But loss of biodiversity is occurring at an alarming rate, and too many livestock are part of the reason.

Biodiversity is undermined by large-scale livestock production in two major ways. The first is deforestation. As discussed in Chapter 2, livestock production is a major impetus for the destruction of forests around the world because the meat sector is constantly seeking more land for pasture and feed-crops. Deforestation reduces wildlife habitat, which threatens animal and plant species. And, once trees are cut down, they are often replaced with single-species monocultures. Then those monocultures get sprayed with pesticides to kill extraneous plants and animals that aren't immediately useful to the short-term economic enterprise.

Industrial meat production also limits biodiversity in another way rarely recognized — by narrowing the livestock gene pool. When many different species and subspecies were employed in agriculture, farm animals were genetically diverse and locally adapted; today's factory farms concentrate on only a few species that have characteristics convenient for mass production.[47] In the 1920s, more than 60 breeds of chicken were raised across the United States, but 21st-century industry relies on just two or three "industrial composite hybrids," says food policy writer Daniel Imhoff.[48] These may be efficient in the short run, but the trend is a serious concern to scientists, farmers, conservationists, and others. For pigs, 15 breeds were raised for the US market about a century ago. Today, at least six of those are extinct, with only three breeds providing three quarters of the genes for commercial pork.[49]

Loss of livestock breeds is dangerous for the same reasons as the loss of any type of food. The trend compromises the ability of communities to produce crops that are suitable to local climate and soil and to employ breeds that are historically and culturally preferable. When fewer species are available, food systems are more vulnerable to changes in conditions—whether it's new pests or new weather patterns. Loss of genetic diversity makes ecosystems less hardy, and it makes livestock less able to resist disease.[50]

In the plant world, for example, tomatoes, carrots, apples, and other crops have been narrowed to a small number of varieties by industrial food systems, as documented by acclaimed author Michael Pollan.[51] Bananas are an example of a rush to specialization.[52] Almost every banana sold in the United States and Canada is now one of those familiar arc-shaped yellow boats called Cavendish, a variety that proved so productive, tasty, and hardy for long-distance transport that it now makes up the vast majority of those fruits imported into North America, and half of those produced worldwide. It's so popular that Americans eat more bananas than any other fresh fruit. But a fungus has been destroying plantations, and the pathogen has been difficult to halt because each Cavendish is genetically identical; bananas no longer have the chromosomal diversity that would make some of them immune to any particular disease agent. As scientists are scrambling to find solutions, the situation serves as a warning against too little diversity in food.[53] The same principle applies to animal-source foods.

But there are rays of hope and islands of commitment to heritage types. For poultry, traditional breeds are making a small, but significant, comeback thanks to a few visionary farmers and groups like Slow Food USA and the American Livestock Breeds Conservancy.[54] Frank Reese Jr., who runs Good Shepherd Poultry in Kansas and who is dedicated to productive, sustainable agriculture, is clear: "The best way to save these historic breeds is to return them to our dinner tables."[55] Mr. Reese has built a business on his belief in diversity, which in animals, as in all of nature, is a basic building block of environmental health.

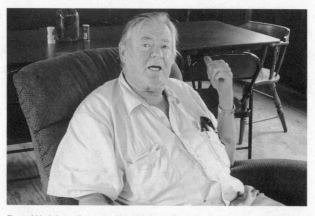

Don Webb, a former North Carolina hog farmer who now opposes CAFOs, says intensive livestock production does not fit with the values most of us hold.

We Want Food Systems to Reflect Our Values

Don Webb of North Carolina, the former hog farmer who now opposes CAFOs, sees intensive livestock farming as just plain wrong. Sitting in his rocking chair on the rural property his family has owned for generations, Mr. Webb talks like a citizen who has done a lot of thinking. He now believes that promoting or even supporting intensive livestock operations is inconsistent with the values of his religion and his country. "It's not Christian," he declares, "and it's not American." Giant pig factories violate basic respect and compassion, he says, and the kinds of rights and freedoms to which we are committed.[56]

Whatever your background and heritage, what Mr. Webb says has the ring of truth. Modern meat systems don't fit with the principles most of us hold, be they religious, spiritual, national, cultural, or just plain common sense. Ultimately, the meat problem raises questions about our values.

To talk about values, we need to talk about the animals. The ethical problems of massive meat production have been documented by others, and are not a major focus of this book. Nevertheless, much of intensive livestock production is a challenge to basic decency and reasonable standards of respect for non-human creatures.[57] Factory-farmed livestock are crowded in small spaces and fed unnaturally dense and medicated diets for fast weight gain. Strongly maternal animals have their babies taken away. Pigs, cows, chickens, and turkeys are subjected to surgical and other painful procedures without anesthetic.[58] Industrial livestock operations deny animals their basic physical, emotional, and social needs.[59] Some of these species are as smart as our beloved dogs, and it has been demonstrated that they possess sentience, the capacity to experience emotion and to suffer.[60] They have nervous systems similar to those of humans, and they possess the anatomy and physiology to feel pleasure and pain.[61]

Most of us feel it is morally acceptable to use animals for some human purposes. But we also hope that chickens, pigs, and cows are not subjected to unnecessary discomfort or suffering. When we eat more meat or buy it more cheaply than can be produced kindly, we violate those hopes. That's why animal-welfare groups disapprove of most intensive production, and it's why organizations such as the Vancouver Humane Society encourage consumers to eat fewer, and more compassionately produced, animal products.[62]

There are critics who believe that even gentle livestock husbandry is wrong, that any meat consumption is unacceptable when humans have other options and the wisdom to make choices. For example, author James McWilliams questions the moral legitimacy of what he calls "happy meat" from livestock raised naturally.[63] But most of us believe it is morally defensible to use animals if we manage them with dignity and a sense of the sacred. The good news is that, if we work toward more sustainable meat systems — low-density livestock numbers in outdoor environments, with few or no chemicals or unnatural feeds — they will also be more compassionate.

Supporters of intensive livestock production argue that animals are better off supervised by people, inside buildings where they are protected from natural predators, and where they are not rooting around in the dirt potentially picking up worms and parasites such as *Trichinella*.[64] It's true that the world can be a dangerous place. But to extend that argument, we'd keep our dogs and cats in cages and our children under lock and key. Natural livestock rancher Joyce Holmes feels differently. She and her family produce sustainable beef at Empire Valley

Ranch in the craggy interior of British Columbia. Their 500-plus cattle live for ten months of the year outdoors "where they are fair game to the predators, but they are in the wide open range."[65] The animals come home to bale grazing for the two coldest months. For Ms. Holmes and similarly minded ranchers, the risk is worth it to produce premium, healthy, grass-fed meat and to do it in a way that has both a history and a future.

Animals aren't the only ones to suffer from intensive production of inexpensive meat; it is also uncompassionate to people. Modern meat systems directly or indirectly make less land available to small farmers around the world. Recall from Chapter 2 that feed crop production uses a full one third of arable land on the planet. Unable to make a living, former smallholders migrate to cities where — especially in developing countries — they often join the urban poor. The imposition of CAFOs on the countryside also ensures that local residents will smell hog barns and experience the decline of country life. Intensive production turns rural work into assembly line jobs with someone else as the boss.

Values are at the center of these issues. The underlying themes have little to do with technicalities or science, but a lot to do with personal and community priorities. We all want sufficient and clean water for life and health. We want a climate that is not destabilized by greenhouse gases. We want antibiotics to work. And most of us want to eat in ways that keep our environment robust, show respect to other creatures, and remain modest in the use of limited resources when a billion people on the planet are hungry.

The topic is often complex, but at the same time it's simple. The issues raised by large-scale meat production and consumption concern compassion, community, and integrity. The meat problem raises questions about the kinds of societies in which we want to live. Whether we think explicitly about values, and whether or not we are religious, most of us have opinions about what is right and wrong and have internal guidelines on how to live. These include treating others with respect and refraining from causing harm. We can transform our food systems as individuals, as communities, and as societies, and in so doing, we can eat and act in ways that reflect our deepest values.

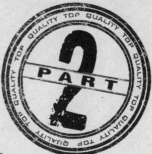

HOW?

STRATEGIES
FOR EATING LESS MEAT

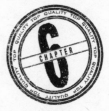

EVERYONE CAN WORK TOWARD
LESS AND BETTER MEAT

It's Perfectly Acceptable to Ask People to Eat Less Meat

Some friends and I were having lunch recently at a downtown restaurant. One of my companions ordered the house salad, but without the chicken. A few minutes later, the server brought a large salad, plus a side plate piled with chicken. "In case you change your mind about the meat," he offered. My friend frowned but didn't send it back, and the flesh food sat untouched until the server came to clean up. "What will happen to the chicken?" someone asked. The server shrugged: "Oh, we'll have to throw it away."

That incident has bothered me for what it says about our attitudes and our food systems. As consumers, we're accustomed to sustenance that is abundant, inexpensive, and disconnected, especially from its animal sources, so it's just more unwanted food. As societies, we make volumes of resource-intensive animal products beyond what people need or even want, then serve it casually and toss it away. The chicken incident suggests to me that we need changes to both production and consumption when it comes to meat. And that's what the science says.

To solve environmental and health problems of livestock, there are only two possible strategies. We can make meat more sustainably, or we can eat less of it. According to a growing pile of reports, we'll need to

99

do both. It's not impossible that third options could arise to allow us to keep making and eating regular servings of meat. For example, there is test-tube meat, a project of the In Vitro Meat Consortium, whose scientists are trying to nurture livestock stem cells to make edible flesh.[1] Other researchers are working on potential large-scale farming of edible insects, species that are already caught in the wild and consumed by two billion people in the developing world.[2] These are fascinating projects, and we'll see how they go. But for the foreseeable future, we need changes to both supply and demand.

"But we just can't ask people to eat less meat!" I've heard this often, from people who say it's draconian and an affront to "personal choice." As one scientific article put it, we need to produce meat more sustainably because "policies directly targeting dietary patterns are often resented as interfering with very personal choices of how and what to eat."[3] One international climate scientist, who I heard interviewed on national radio, laid out powerful evidence of environmental devastation from large-scale meat production and consumption. But when asked whether consumers shouldn't eat less meat, the scientist spluttered: "Oh, we can't ask them to do that. People have a right to eat as they choose."

In my opinion, this stance just isn't logical. First, food educators constantly recommend that people change their eating habits to consume more fruits and vegetables, and food activists urge people to eat local. No one seems to be offended by these suggestions to eat more, so they shouldn't really be offended by suggestions to eat less, even of our beloved meat.

Second, societies regularly mandate that people rein in short-term desires for the common good, and most of us comply, knowing that others will too. We follow traffic rules and pay our taxes, recognizing that human rights require balance between our wishes as individuals and the wishes of others and the community.

There is a third reason it is morally acceptable to recommend that people eat less meat. Our societies already play a powerful role in people's food choices — in the case of meat, by supporting and encouraging intensive production, as we will see in Chapter 8. Governments already influence our "personal choice," so they might as well do so in ways that are healthy for the environment and for us.[4]

But the "eat less meat" suggestion can bring out the libertarian in people. Boris Johnson, the idiosyncratic mayor of London, England, is one example. Incensed by a prominent scientist's proposal that people limit their consumption, Mr. Johnson wrote a newspaper article proclaiming "the whole proposition is so irritating that I am almost minded to eat more meat in response."[5] The mayor is not alone in bristling at the recommendation. Producers and retailers are, in some cases, on the offense, and industry supporters have established an annual Meat-In Day at Penn State University in response to the Great American Meat-Out Day.[6] The debate can get heated. One Australian professor suggested that eating vegetarian meals gives you "animal blood on your hands."[7] As he argues, eating plants requires farming that endangers mice and other creatures, while red meat can be produced on grassland that isn't good for much else. He's probably correct that grazing livestock is an optimal use of some rangelands, but most meat eaten in the United States and Canada required large amounts of land for feed, so it's unlikely that vegetarians kill more animals than do meat-eaters. But it's all part of the global discussion taking place, as we figure out what constitutes sustainable consumption.

People who live in rural areas with easy access to good animal products may well be able to keep consuming them regularly. One rancher I interviewed believes that people can eat meat often when it is grown sustainably, like her family does. She adds that our environments contain a myriad of pollutants and drugs, so that any ill effects of meat are small in comparison.[8]

It's going to take time, and more research, to sort out how much can be produced and consumed without excessive greenhouse gases, pollution, and ill health. Until then, the science suggests that — especially for urbanites whose steaks, chicken, and ribs come largely from factory farms[9] — cutting back significantly will help make food systems tenable for the long term.

Everyone Can Be Involved in This Project

The first half of this book outlined reasons to tackle the meat problem. Now let's turn to strategies: top-down or supply-related improvements to production, and bottom-up or demand-related improvements to consumption. Because both will be needed, we can all be part of the project.

Scientists and producers are working on technical and management strategies for making meat with fewer resources and less waste, and those kinds of improvements will be essential.[10] *Livestock's Long Shadow* co-authors Henning Steinfeld and Pierre Gerber believe "there is a vast mitigation potential on the production side," with careful use of technology and intensification.[11] The topic is climbing on the agenda of producers, researchers, and policymakers. Sustainability is now a regular topic at conferences and meetings on livestock and meat, and key organizations are bringing high-level researchers and policy experts together to hammer out ideas on meeting human protein needs more ecologically than we're doing today.[12]

But even if producers do their best, improvements to current systems are unlikely to suffice. According to one widely quoted analysis, production improvements may only decrease livestock-related greenhouse gases by about 25%, and overall livestock-derived pollution and health problems by about 20%.[13] That's good, but not good enough, considering the threat of climate change and the health dangers of water contamination and environmental degradation. Heavy meat consumption just takes too great an ecological toll, even today, let alone at the higher levels projected for the next few decades.[14] Researchers have crunched the numbers and concluded that we'll also need to lower our consumption.[15] Environmental scientists Nathan Pelletier and Peter Tyedmers of Dalhousie University suggest strongly that government policy should help citizens decrease their consumption.[16] And, according to the Washington-based Environmental Working Group, no matter how "greenly" we produce meat, we'll still need to eat less of it.[17]

"Even if every tool in the box were thrown at lowering emissions from livestock production, we would fail to cut our footprint as far as we need," according to European researchers who brought together industry and other stakeholders to develop solutions to meat-induced climate change. They concluded that better production is essential, but so are consumption shifts.[18]

Climate-change expert and former US Vice President Al Gore has said that eating less meat is important to fight global warming and other environmental problems. "I'm not a vegetarian," he said in a television interview, "but I have cut back sharply on the meat that I eat, and it's absolutely correct that the growing meat intensity of diets around the world is one of the issues connected to this global crisis."[19] American health experts, including Dr. Barry Popkin, have shown that reductions in meat consumption would have strong and multiple benefits for the environment and health.[20]

Supply and demand are intertwined, of course, so that changes to one affect the other. If large numbers of people stop buying factory-farmed meat in favor of local, ecologically raised chicken and beef, the change would get noticed by industry, which would buckle down and figure out ways to expand sustainable production. That's what's happening with organic foods, a fast-developing segment in agriculture and grocery. As well, influence can occur in the opposite direction, with supply affecting demand. Now that more leading-edge ranchers and farmers are producing sustainable meat, more consumers will become amenable to paying the higher prices for better food.

Just as supply and demand are intertwined, so are they tied to policy — that mesh of laws, regulations, and customs set by governments and other actors. Policy sets the stage for supply and demand, helping determine what foods get made (and how) and what retail choices are available. Authorities decide what kinds of agriculture to encourage. They design tax structures and offer farm assistance programs, which give a push to some kinds of food production more than others.[21] The US Farm Bill has had enormous effect on food supply and demand. Daniel Imhoff, whose book *Food Fight* deconstructs the legislation, suggests it too often facilitates corporate control of food and invites bad eating. Mr. Imhoff and other analysts say the bill bears responsibility for a system in which most children have unhealthy diets, much of Americans' vegetable intake consists of potato chips and fries, and Americans are beset with obesity and diabetes.[22]

Policy influences production, but also consumption. When you and I shop for groceries, we may feel we're exercising personal preferences. Yet our choices are constrained by laws, regulations, and policy priorities. Breakfast cereals, for example, appear to offer diversity and selection, but it's an illusion of choice. Multiple brands of processed cereals are often made by just a few companies. Ingredients are similar from one box to the next, and most contain unnecessary sweeteners. Similarly, animal-source foods appear to offer options. But, especially in large chain stores, most of the pork and beef being sold came off production lines and was trucked in from a factory farm run by one of a handful of companies. Remember that one reason people eat so much meat today is because it has often been priced below the true cost of production. Government priorities have made it so, by promoting mass production, by subsidizing feedstuffs, and by failing to require that producers pay the full costs of cleanup.

If meat were produced in real market conditions, retail prices would increase and consumption would probably decrease. How much less people would eat if prices were higher would depend on several factors: on consumer perceptions of how necessary meat is (or is not); on the edible substitutes that are available (and that consumers are willing to try); and on whether people have (or have not) figured out how to cook plant-based meals. We'll talk more about potential government tactics and their consequences in Chapter 8. But it is clear that policy can directly affect consumer behavior.[23] And it is also clear that government has the ability to change food systems in a way that can still provide appealing choices to the consumer.

One way policy can affect consumption is through recommendations. In San Francisco and in Washington, DC, city officials have passed resolutions supporting the international movement Meatless Monday.[24] These cities have joined a list of other communities and individuals to promote the idea of going meatless one day out of seven. Other cities that have adopted Meatless Monday include Aspen, Colorado; Durham/Raleigh, North Carolina; and Covington, Kentucky.[25]

In Belgium, the city of Ghent has initiated Veggie Day, suggesting residents forgo meat on Thursdays, for the good of the environment. Meatless Monday and similar campaigns have caught on and are being promoted by individuals, chefs, restaurants, the media, and public health organizations.[26] Baltimore and other school districts have signed on, as have universities from California to Florida.[27] More than 20 countries now have groups actively promoting Meatless Monday. In Cincinnati, Ohio, a 2008 Climate Protection Action Plan suggested the city recommend "reduced consumption of meat in individual and institutional diets."[28] It's too early to tell how large an effect such suggestions will have, but such widespread involvement is a promising sign.

Recommending sustainable consumption can be an uphill battle with a steep grade, as Sweden found out. Its National Food Agency published draft guidelines in 2009 suggesting environmentally friendly dietary choices for its citizens, including more local foods and fewer animal products.[29] This might seem ecologically sensible. But the European Union scolded Sweden for recommending that consumers buy food produced at home rather than that produced in other countries. According to the EU, such recommendations contravene the letter and spirit of trade agreements,[30] and by 2011, Sweden had withdrawn the guidelines.[31] Those guidelines had boldly raised the meat issue on page one, citing beef, lamb, pork, and chicken as foodstuffs with the worst environmental impact. "To eat less meat, and to choose what you eat with care, is therefore the most effective environmental choice you can make."[32] Now the country has published the supporting information on a website,[33] but with none of the recommendations for citizens, who will need to figure it out for themselves.

Much of the scuffle concerns trade agreements, the World Trade Organization system of liberalized exchange of goods and lowered barriers to international business. Even if the United States and Canada wanted to stop encouraging factory farms and start supporting local sustainable livestock production, trade agreements would make it difficult. This is the case despite widespread criticism that free trade is built on questionable assumptions, such as ongoing access to affordable fossil fuels. Critics of the prevailing trade model say it undermines the environment by sanctioning excessive energy use for transportation and by making it difficult for countries to implement environmental standards. It reminds me of that economics maxim that there's no such thing as a free lunch. When goods and services are provided, some-one — somewhere — pays. This is also true for global agreements mandating long-distance consumption. Someone or something pays, and often that something is the environment, suggesting there's no such thing as a free trade.

Opponents of healthy dietary guidelines also reared their heads in England in 2009. The National Health Service had suggested that hospitals serve less meat as part of a carbon reduction strategy. But that was widely interpreted as a ban on meat, and the government plan was scrapped.[34] In Australia, there are furious debates over whether the government's dietary guidelines and food policy will have a sustainability dimension. The Public Health Association of Australia argues that it should,[35] but parts of the food industry disagree.

So it won't be a cakewalk, which is a good reason for all of us to get involved. And because we need changes to both supply and demand, for which public policy will be required, whole societies can help face the meat problem. The project will require commitment from the bottom up by consumers and citizens, and from the top down by policymakers and corporations. The meat problem is a project that can be addressed by everyone, whatever their relationship to meat and whatever their politics. Whether we call ourselves vegetarians or carnivores, we're all omnivores,[36] and we all have the same planet to save. Farmer and urbanite, environmentalist and business executive, are all concerned about water quality, climate stability, and human well-being. Nor should the meat problem and the environmental challenges of factory farming be progressive or left-wing political issues. Conservative and liberal, religious and secular, are concerned about kindness and dignity for people and animals. Joel Salatin is a vocal opponent of industrial farming who is neither a "rural hayseed or neo-hippie,"[37] but a social conservative with strong religious faith and libertarian economic views. Owner of Polyface Farm in Virginia, Mr. Salatin recommends that we stop accepting industrial animal products and other foods as the norm, and instead make our meals local and sustainable. Another who argues against intensive meat production is author and Republican Party speech writer Matthew Scully. In his "case for compassionate conservatism," Mr. Scully appeals to so-called right-wingers as well as to the left, saying industrial meat factories violate the moral teachings of every faith and the "widely shared principles" of us all.[38]

Livestock producers need to be part of the solution, and in some cases, they already are. But the industry has felt alienated from discussions about meat and the environment — and unfairly blamed. Ranchers and agribusiness executives may not feel enthusiastic about joining an "eat less meat" movement. But they care about environmental and community issues, and many (if partly in the name of doing good business) will want to be involved as this topic gains profile. Producers are on a treadmill that's fueled by the pressure for low retail prices. Yet some are sincerely interested in creating food systems that can deliver decent financial returns to farmers, especially small to moderate-sized sustainable ones. Ideally, producers will work with citizens for solutions. Our common sense, our compassion, and our desire for environmental and personal health suggest we can all be part of this project.

Meat Can Be Made More Sustainably

Mike Williams has a report on his desk showing five different ways of dramatically lessening pollution from livestock waste. They're newly engineered ways of dealing with large volumes of manure, and all have been identified as Environmentally Superior Technologies for the intensive swine industry. The report, published in 2006, demonstrated how these new technologies can lower hog pollution by 25–50%.[39] Since then, however, only about a dozen producers out of 2,000 in the state have signed on. That's less than 1%. The vast majority continue to use the method of storing and treating manure in open lagoons and spraying it as fertilizer on farmland.

Dr. Williams knows the report well, since he wrote it himself, part of his 20 years of work on these topics. Professor and director of the North Carolina State University Animal and Poultry Waste Management

Center, he headed a detailed series of studies to assess new manure-management systems for hogs.[40]

Like many environmentally friendly systems, these manure management technologies require a significant investment. Each one costs up to half a million dollars to install, then operating costs can be several times higher than existing methods. Meat producers would rather not pay, and governments don't insist on it. But Dr. Williams is disappointed at the low uptake and frustrated at the lack of cost-sharing and other government incentives. Environmentally friendly systems can't really be fine-tuned until designers get feedback that allows for the iterative process of technological improvement. And until that happens, costs won't go down. But most livestock operations are sticking with current methods.

Better manure management is one way to make meat with less pollution and fewer greenhouse gases, and many researchers are working on additional ideas. For example, beef producers can be part of the solution if cattle are pastured in ways that minimize emissions of methane and nitrous oxide.[41] Certain kinds of forage (e.g., those containing more legumes) are easier to digest and therefore make for less methane. Some land management strategies are more climate-friendly than others, such as avoiding blanket use of nitrogen fertilizers and keeping animal densities low. Then there are ways to reduce gaseous emissions from fertilizers, to capture and use methane, and to otherwise persuade livestock to leave a smaller ecological footprint.[42]

Smithfield Foods, the world's largest pork producer, is aware of the issues. I had a lengthy phone interview with Dennis Treacy, vice president and chief sustainability officer for the Virginia-based company.[43] Mr. Treacy's office has a growing stack of books written by people who don't like corporate food systems. But few of the researchers inquired after the company's point of view, he said, so they were happy to be asked. Mr. Treacy conceded that the hog industry has caused environmental problems, especially in the early years when farms were not run to modern standards. But Smithfield is working to produce pork more in line with ecosystems, he said. They're working on cleaning up waste and finding channels for it, such as using it to generate energy. And they're decreasing their use of water and energy, as is stated in the list of sustainability commitments on their website.[44]

But producers have financial goals and constraints, and observers outside the industry say companies are unlikely to take big leaps toward sustainability unless new practices are also made compulsory for their competitors. Professor Pete Smith, climate change scientist at the University of Aberdeen, and his colleagues have said greenhouse gases in farming could be markedly decreased. Yet "despite significant biophysical potential for GHG mitigation in agriculture, very little progress has been made since 1990,"[45] and not a lot can be expected without policy changes. Solutions aren't solutions until they're implemented.

The system is crying out for a more informed public policy—to rationalize livestock systems, to set and enforce tough environmental standards, and to ensure that rules and regulations don't discriminate against independent producers. In the long run, policy will need to take a bolder view. That's the view of J. P. Reganold, agricultural scientist at the University of Washington, and his co-authors, who called in 2011 for both "incremental and transformative" changes to food systems.[46] Incremental tactics, like better crop rotation, are important. But we also need to imagine deep shifts that would fully integrate agriculture and livestock into ecosystems.

Social Systems Can Change. People Can Change

It's hard to imagine wholesale changes to agriculture and food. But history is full of examples of social innovations that were initially derided as impossible and unacceptable. Human slavery was legal not so long ago.[47] When opponents argued for abolition, they were up against supporters of the status quo who argued that the economy was based on slave labor and that abolition would be disruptive and destabilizing. That may have been true, but that argument wasn't good enough then, and it wouldn't be good enough now. Other powerful social shifts have included the extension of voting rights to women and, more recently, public acceptance for gay rights. These issues and others were once controversial, but are widely supported today.

There are many small, but significant, examples. Car seatbelts, in my part of the world, have only been mandatory for a few decades. I remember debates on whether seatbelt use should be compulsory, and protests from opponents that such laws would violate individual rights. But the pro-seatbelt arguments won out, and today most people just buckle up. A more dramatic example involves smoking. In my region, it wasn't long ago that people smoked anywhere and everywhere. When citizens started discussing potential limits to public smoking, debates were emotional. Some people protested that limits would abrogate smokers' rights. Since then, the majority has come to feel that non-smokers have rights too, and in only a few years, social norms on this issue have changed so utterly that almost no one objects when smokers are forced to stand in the freezing rain for a puff. An additional example concerns what dogs leave behind. In my town, when I was a child, dog waste lay in neighborhood parks, on sidewalks, and at street curbs. Today a municipal bylaw requires that dog-owners clean up after their pets. The change didn't happen overnight, but it happened, and today the community is cleaner and healthier. Turning societies around takes time and effort. But social change can and does take hold.

Individuals can also change. Where meat is concerned, some say they already have. "We hardly eat any meat these days," I've been told. "We eat much less meat than we used to." At first I thought people were engaging in little friendly exaggeration to make my day, but there is, indeed, a trend. There are signs of it in North America,[48] though some European countries are ahead of us. A recent poll in the Netherlands showed that well over half of consumers identify themselves as "meat reducers" who are voluntarily restricting their consumption.[49] Eating less meat is a shift that — in small ways — is already occurring, as noted on the food site epicurious.com[50] and shown by market researchers.[51]

Nevertheless, there persists a belief that people are incapable of cutting back on their meat consumption. Maybe it's the raw lust evoked by the idea of meat, which is odd since no one would accept that it's impossible to control other kinds of lust. It may be a statement of hope from those who like their culinary habits. The belief that heavy meat-eating

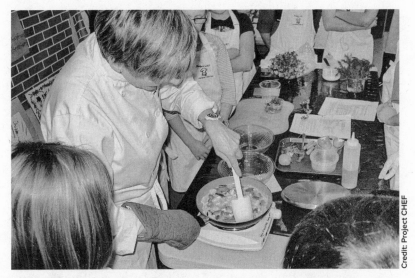

Cooking is fun and can be delicious with a maximum of plant-based ingredients and a minimum of animal products. That's the lesson from Project CHEF (Cook Healthy Edible Food) and its food teachers like Barb Finley, here, surrounded by children.

is intractable may also be tied to the widely held myth that people can't change.

Altering behavior can indeed be difficult, especially habits that are as tied to culture, family, and identity as those involving food. Desire can be powerful for meatballs the way your mother used to make them. But that doesn't mean you need meatballs — or any meat — every day.

The truth is, as the psychological literature demonstrates, people are capable of significantly changing their ways. A heavy drinker stops imbibing and takes charge of his life. A dangerous driver slows down, and a busy mother stops using her cell phone while driving, each after near-accidents. An overweight person musters the courage of control, especially following the positive reinforcement of weight loss. People alter their behavior when sufficiently motivated to do so. That's the general rule in psychology, and it applies to habits and life patterns of many kinds. People can change when they have compelling arguments and practical strategies for doing so. In other words, they need good reasons and a plan.

We've got reasons to eat less meat, and we're capable of creating a plan. We know meat isn't necessary every day, and just need ways of acting on that knowledge. We need to break old habits and develop new ones and find different ways of shopping for food and preparing and eating it. We can do this without the sanction of political or bureaucratic structures, but simply our own heads and hands. Food represents a perfect opportunity for consumers to lower their personal footprint because of food's dramatic environmental impact, and because we make many choices about food every day.[52]

Individuals can have power, especially in the absence of potent political structures, for solving dilemmas as enmeshed as the meat problem. For massive human challenges — think war or climate change — global political mechanisms are sometimes unable to find solutions. For that reason, improving food systems will partly be facilitated through grassroots action. As one group of experts wrote about livestock and meat: "In a global economy, with no global society, it may well be up to consumers to set a sustainable course."[53]

How Much Less?

Less than half of what we now eat.

That's the short version of how much meat the average American and Canadian may be able to consume for sustainability and health. It's essentially an expert guess from scientists, who say it's not possible to be more precise. But whether they're figuring out how to stabilize livestock emissions, get water pollution under control, or mitigate health problems from excessive consumption, numerous experts have suggested we trim our intake to roughly half of what most of us now eat.

Environmentally, how much animal-source consumption is justifiable — now, let alone in the future — depends on many factors: the degree to which we can minimize greenhouse gas emissions and pollution from other sources; how much conservation of water and other resources can successfully be applied to livestock production; and where and how you live. The suggestion to significantly lower your meat consumption won't necessarily apply if you raise your own animals and eat more in tune with nature than urbanites who don't grow their own. But in general, most people may need to cut their meat intake from a few times a day to a few times a week.

There are no rules on this, and no requirement that you comply. But if you want to be part of this environmental project, consume less often or in smaller amounts. You can have a little more if it's chicken, a little less if it's red meat. It is possible to eat red meat and still call yourself an environmentalist if you limit it to small and occasional portions. Go ahead and have a small amount of dairy each day and fish each week, especially if they are from sustainable sources.

The benchmark McMichael study, "Food, Livestock Production, Energy, Climate Change, and Health," calls for residents in high-intake countries like the United States and Canada to cut their meat consumption to levels that would put a lid on livestock emissions.[54] To do that, we'd need to decrease our intake about 60%, from 200–250 grams (about 7–9 ounces) per person per day, down to less than 90 grams (about 3 ounces), with no more than 50 grams (less than 2 ounces) of that from red meat. That study, introduced in Chapter 2, assumes that citizens of developing countries will continue to increase their meat intake from roughly 50 grams per person per day. It also assumes world population will continue to rise, which will intensify the meat-and-environment challenge. On the other side of the ledger is the understanding that the meat sector will improve production methods and lower livestock-related methane and nitrous oxide by up to 20%.[55]

The McMichael report has been misquoted as recommending we should lower our meat consumption by 10%, a confusion that arose because the report called for a worldwide cutback from the current international average of 100 grams (3.5 ounces) per person per day to 90 grams. But today's 100-gram average intake is for the planet as a whole, while we in industrialized countries take in more than twice that much. For those of us living in wealthy nations, the overt recommendation is for a decrease of considerably more than half. As well, under this plan, daily per capita consumption of red meat should be less than 50 grams. That's less than half of one quarter-pound burger, so you could — at most — eat one of those every second day, if you want to get on board.

Cornell University scientists David and Marcia Pimentel have been writing for years about the powerful need for reductions in animal-source foods, and they agree we should halve our meat and dairy as part of overall changes in eating patterns.[56] They also promote less overall caloric intake, less junk food, and more locally produced meals, contending that such diets provide plenty of nutrients and are beneficial for health.[57]

Other health researchers warn against eating — on a daily basis — even a single quarter-pound burger, or one small steak, or one pork chop, or four bacon slices. Those amounts would put you in the "high consumption" category that makes you more vulnerable to cancer. As discussed in Chapter 4, researchers at the National Institutes of Health showed that high consumers of red and processed meats are more likely to develop colorectal and other cancers.[58] I asked lead investigator Amanda Cross what they called high consumption, and she itemized it as listed above, starting with one quarter-pound burger a day.[59] Happily, the statistical associations between regular meat consumption and cancer are what scientists call "dose-response," meaning they're dependent on amounts. While regular large servings may increase your vulnerability, small ones basically won't.

So how much meat can you eat for health? It depends on a lot of factors, but the World Cancer Research Fund and the American Institute for Cancer Research have suggested that people who eat red meat keep their weekly intake to less than 18 ounces — a maximum of just over a pound every seven days — with very little of it processed.[60] So you could eat the equivalent of four quarter-pound burgers a week, if that was all the red meat you ate. For most of us, it's food for thought.

A "Fair, Less Meat Diet" is a suggestion from European researchers that would provide enough protein but allow animal products to be farmed better and distributed more equitably. Following this diet plan, consumers would obtain most of their protein from non-animal sources and eat meat 2 or 3 times a week, with some dairy each day.[61] This idea emerged from research by non-governmental organizations Friends of the Earth and Compassion in World Farming.[62] The latter group has long promoted the reform of meat and dairy production and consumption, and has suggested reductions of even 60% or more below current levels by 2050.[63] Environmental commentator Jonathon Porritt doubts that 50% cuts will suffice, and underscores that decreasing consumption to 90 grams a day (about 3 ounces) will, at best, stabilize livestock greenhouse gas emissions at 2005 levels. "But no need to scare the horses at this stage, let alone eat them," he writes, so we'll go with that.[64] Deeper cuts may indeed be needed, but for now, a good target is for 50% less meat consumption for the US, Canada, the UK, and other high-intake parts of the world.

Any decrease would help, given the seriousness of the relevant environmental and health issues. Because of that, we can look to useful campaigns such as Meatless Monday — not just for encouraging people to forgo meat one day a week, but for demonstrating that meals don't need to include animal products to be satisfying and delicious. Some activists have promoted the concept of the "Weekday Vegetarian," recommending people eat meat on weekends only.[65] Such campaigns will need some strong social media and marketing genius to make them something everybody wants to do.[66]

It may sound naïve to imagine that whole populations could cut back significantly on their meat intake. But the unthinkable is becoming thinkable. Scientists have known for years about the environmental burden of intensive large-scale meat production, yet have assumed consumers won't cut back. "Substantial voluntary reductions of meat consumption are not very likely,"[67] said prominent scientist Vaclav Smil in 2002. But his latest book, *Eating Meat*, slated for publication in 2012, outlines the environmental necessity for what he calls "rational meat eating," which would include fewer animal products and more sustainable production. Naïve we may be, but action is imperative. With hope and cooperation, we can work toward lowering the stakes.

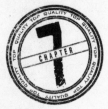

PEOPLE CAN MODERATE
THEIR CONSUMPTION

Take It from a Chef

Helping people eat less meat is what Annie Somerville does. She's the renowned executive chef at Greens, the San Francisco restaurant that is one of the best-known meatless eating spots in North America. The restaurant is often full, and not just with vegetarians, since the majority of Greens' customers are at least occasional meat-eaters. Though Ms. Somerville doesn't have statistics, she's been chatting with Greens' customers for 30 years. She says diners love the food because it is tasty, beautiful, and healthy.

Ms. Somerville exemplifies the trend to relaxing the line between vegetarians and meat-eaters and concentrating on eating healthier overall. She cooks only vegetarian cuisine, using dairy products, but no meat or fish. Personally, she occasionally eats a small piece of fish if it's wild and fresh, or chicken if it is sustainably produced. "I'm not stringent about it, but am vegetarian most of the time."[1]

Her advice for people wanting to eat less meat is to ease into it. "Make it a gradual transition," she counsels. Make it a real transformation and not just a crash diet that won't last. "We're all creatures of habit, but we can shift."

As a food expert, Ms. Somerville is concerned that people don't cook enough and rely instead on processed and prepared foods. She's

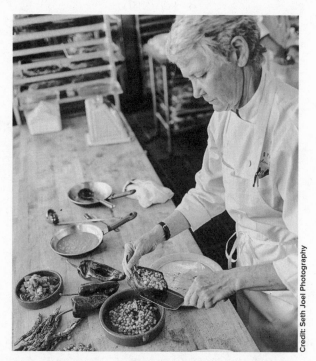

Credit: Seth Joel Photography

Annie Somerville, executive chef at Greens restaurant in San Francisco, prepares tasty and nutritious meatless meals.

concerned that people consume too many sodas rather than what she considers the best drink: water. (That's what she regularly drinks, with a twist of lemon or mint.) She's concerned that people expect food to be inexpensive, although they readily pay for non-necessities. She's concerned that governments don't sufficiently support small agriculture. She's concerned that Americans are "a terrible influence on people around the world who can't afford a giant piece of animal protein on their plates."

But Ms. Somerville is optimistic about consumer interest in good food. From her weekly visits to the local farmers' market, and from the enthusiasm of Greens' customers, she sees modern food culture as "vigorous" and "electric." As part of this new awareness, more and more people are talking about political, environmental, and social reasons to cut back on their meat intake.

We Can Be Personal Agents of Change

We can't always rely on policymakers to lead us toward sustainable production (as we've seen in past chapters). So, too, we can't necessarily rely on health professionals to lead us toward optimal consumption. Even clinical experts often respond to syndromes such as high cholesterol not by recommending dietary shifts, but by prescribing medications. Patients can be reluctant to change their diets, and pharmaceuticals have their place. But if we're going to solve the meat problem, we'll need to change our diets, and we'll need to make that decision ourselves.

We can each become agents of change for the environment, for health, and for global well-being. And we can start today.[2] One advantage to consumer action is that it can start immediately, without meetings or legislation. We, as individuals, can help solve the meat problem by making new choices for this evening's meal and by supporting restaurants and retailers that understand the significance of the issue.

We can also propel the "eat less meat" movement beyond our personal choices, by getting involved in citizen groups. There are effective non-governmental organizations targeting climate change, water pollution, and other issues related to industrial meat, including antibiotics and other chemicals in animal agriculture. Our communities all have organizations promoting animal welfare and educating people to eat lower on the food chain. Some of these groups are listed in Appendix II and on the website and Facebook page of this book.

Whether working alone, with friends and neighbors, or through organizations, we have the ability to write letters and raise issues, through social media or conventional channels, any of which can create ripple effects. We have the option to communicate with elected officials, urging them to support local, small-scale organic livestock producers rather than factory farms. When top-down systems are stuck in a mire of special interests and administrative paralysis, citizens can take action from the bottom up.

But why should we take personal action when others don't? What about China? I've been asked why citizens in North America should do the work and make the sacrifice to decrease their intake of animal products when hundreds of millions in middle-income nations are rapidly increasing theirs. It's true that in developing and emerging countries per capita meat consumption has more than doubled since 1980, and per-person intake of milk and eggs has also soared. China is a dramatic example. Since 1980, per capita consumption of meat has quadrupled, consumption of milk has increased by tenfold, and intake of eggs has increased eightfold.[3] That's despite a history of little dairy consumption in China, where many people are lactose intolerant.[4] By 2050, when the world is projected to have 9 billion people, per capita meat consumption in developing and emerging nations is predicted to increase even more.[5]

People around the world are indeed embracing animal products. Nevertheless, residents of China, India, Africa, and most of Latin America still consume much less, per capita, than do we in the United States, Canada, and Europe.[6] Even by 2050, the average person in the developing world is projected to consume fewer animal products than the average person in the industrialized world.[7] We, in the West, are the main problem and are therefore in the strongest position to make a difference. We also have access to a wide variety of nutritious and delicious foods other than solely meats, dairy, and fish.

Besides, authorities and researchers worldwide are aware of the need to mitigate negative consequences of soaring meat consumption. In Beijing, a Sustainable Agriculture Innovation Network (SAIN) is hosted by the Chinese Academy of Agricultural Sciences.[8] British researchers went to Beijing in 2011 for partnership meetings with SAIN, and attendee Basia Romanowicz of the World Society for the Protection of Animals told me later there is growing interest among Chinese officials and researchers for sustainability and animal welfare in meat production.[9] Food activists and environmentalists in poor countries are also working on these issues. In India, scientists such as Dr. Vandana Shiva are promoting locally controlled agriculture and food production that can provide for all citizens of one of the most populous nations on Earth.[10] There are no good excuses for us as individuals, the world's highest per capita meat consumers, to avoid taking initiative in being agents of change.

We Can Develop New Attitudes and Strategies

"Meat-less" eating is more a state of mind than a set of skills. It's based on attitudes and strategies that we can develop for planning meals, shopping for groceries, and preparing food. Here are a few places to start.

Remember that we can prepare desirable
and delicious meals with a minimum of animal products.

There's a considerable variety of grains, legumes, vegetables, and fruits out there, many of which you may never have tried. It helps to rethink beliefs, especially ones formed long ago, about what foods are desirable. Steak and chicken breast may sound sophisticated, but carrots, beans, lentils, and leafy greens are cultured cuisine of a different kind.

You don't have to give up delicious food for meatless meals. There's a myth that vegetarian food is bland, but people who say this often douse their meat in ketchup, salt, and pepper. In many cases, it's not the food we taste, but the condiments. But if you enjoy it, there's no rule that says you can't use a little barbecue sauce on sautéed vegetables and rice.

The perception that plant-based food is dull deserves comment from a scientific perspective. Humans are genetically programmed to seek high-calorie sustenance with sugars and fats. Meat qualifies. So it's true that flesh foods contain an ingredient that inherently appeals to the human palate. But we can satisfy and train our palate with meatless meals, using vegetable oils along with foods that are naturally sweet. Vegetarian meals can be exquisitely tasty.

Recognize that preparing plant-based meals can be done
with little extra time and effort. Meal plans and
ingredients can be straightforward.

It's 5 PM, you've already had a full day, and your family members are wondering what's for dinner and how soon. How can you find the time to do something different from usual?

Eating less meat does require adjustment. However, once you've started making the change, food preparation doesn't need to be complicated. There are more vegetables to chop, but the food processor helps.

And there are other shortcuts you can take, such as using canned beans, rather than dry.

You don't need fancy ingredients. You don't even need "meat substitutes" — processed alternatives such as vegetarian ham and sausage, though these can be convenient and tasty. Try to increase your intake of a broad base of fresh plant foods and simple cereals.

You'll find specific tips in Appendix I, which give you ideas on lowering your meat consumption without spending much extra time in planning or preparation. You'll also find simple recipes for everyday dishes my family makes. And there's a special recipe direct from Greens executive chef Annie Somerville.

Plan to use animal products frugally, and waste less.

Decreasing wastage of meat, dairy, and fish is powerful action each of us can take. The sad truth is that considerable amounts of animal-source foods never get eaten, but go straight to the landfill. Uneaten meat can account for 20% of the greenhouse gases associated with producing, processing, transporting, and consuming animal products.[11] Food waste is unsupportable in the face of chronic hunger for hundreds of millions of global citizens. But waste is especially tragic in the case of animal products, which required so much of the Earth's resources — and so much sacred animal life — to produce.[12]

To minimize waste, buy right-sized portions rather than excess. Don't dispose of animal leftovers, but refrigerate them and find a creative way to whip them into something different the next day.

Help the industry decrease waste by "eating the whole animal," which means buying unusual meat cuts, rather than only ones considered choice. Support restaurants that do the same. There are increasing numbers of dining establishments that serve pork belly, beef heart, and other bits.[13] It's a revival of a frugal style from past generations, and it's not only conservationist, it's chic.[14]

Find sources of sustainable meat.

Seek out places to buy the best kinds of animal products — from livestock that were raised naturally, rather than solely on concentrated feeds; that didn't regularly receive antibiotics, hormones, or other chemicals; that lived mostly outdoors; and that were raised on locally owned ranches and farms. Such sources are increasingly available. Nevertheless, it may take persistence. Dietician and food professor Marion Nestle went to supermarkets looking for organic meat, and she had trouble finding the real thing. What she did find were stacks of meat labeled "natural," a hopeful-sounding term, but not a very meaningful one.[15] While some terms including "organic" are strictly defined and enforced, many others, including "natural," are less well-defined and are "often misused on labels and in advertisements."[16] Look for good meats at your local grocery stores, but also look for other sources including Community Supported Agriculture (CSA) organizations.[17]

If meat is certified organic, it satisfies strict rules for raising livestock with minimal chemicals, processing, preservatives, or artificial ingredients,[18] but if not certified organic, it may still adhere to high standards. "Certified Local Sustainable" is an eco-label from the Toronto-based Local Food Plus (LFP) that takes into account an impressive array of social, ecological, and ethical factors. LFP certifies farmers and processors who (get ready for a mouthful): reduce synthetic pesticides and fertilizers; avoid hormones, antibiotics, and genetic engineering; conserve soil and water; provide safe and fair working conditions for farm labor; provide healthy and humane care for livestock; protect and enhance wildlife habitat and biodiversity on farm landscapes; and reduce energy consumption and greenhouse gas emissions.[19] There are other welfare and eco-labels to look for, including Certified Humane[20] and American Welfare Approved.[21]

Be willing to pay more than you would for conventional beef, chicken, or pork.

Once we find better meat, we need to be willing to pay what it's worth. That's hard, since we've become accustomed to relatively low food prices. North Americans spend only about 10% of their disposable incomes on food, while Europeans spend more than 20% of theirs, and two billion of the poorest global citizens spend 50–70% of their incomes on food.[22] This all sounds as if Americans and Canadians are fortunate.

But inexpensive food—particularly from the meat department—can harm the planet and our health. As well-known food writer Michael Pollan points out, most of us could afford to spend more on food if we valued it. Meanwhile, as we spend less and less on food, we spend more and more to treat our illnesses. Fifty years ago, Americans spent 18% of their incomes on food and 5% on health care, yet today spend only 10% of their incomes on food but 16% on health care.[23] It's difficult to believe this is a coincidence.

While low food prices may seem like a treat, they're really a trap. A chicken-industry consultant once told me that producers would like to use more ecological methods. "But there's one big problem. Customers don't want to pay much for food." Livestock and meat companies could concentrate more on quality if consumers would concentrate less on price.

The good stuff usually does cost more. The price premium on sustainably and compassionately raised meat can range anywhere from just a fraction more to several times the price of conventional meat. The other day, I phoned a nearby Whole Foods, where rib-eye steak was selling for two to three times the price of the factory-farmed rib-eye at a mainstream grocer nearby. But Whole Foods carries only meat from livestock raised without hormones or antibiotics under the 5-Step Animal-Welfare guidelines from the Global Animal Partnership,[24] a non-profit organization committed to improving conditions for animals in food production. Many other retailers carry sustainable animal products, but make sure you check the labels to know what you are getting.

The heartening news is that price is not consumers' only consideration. Whole Foods chief executive, John Mackey, has witnessed this in his 30-plus years at the leading natural foods retailer. While some shoppers just want low prices, his company has discovered "that people are increasingly willing to spend more to get higher quality-food. Food from more responsible, more sustainable, and more ethical farms."[25] One survey showed that Canadian consumers are, at least in theory, willing to pay more for compassionately produced food. In two successive years, almost three quarters of respondents said they would agree to higher prices for farm animal products certified to humane standards of care by a third party.[26] International data backs this up, showing that discerning middle-income consumers will pay more if they have enough information to believe that higher-priced foods are safer or otherwise superior.[27]

"Values for money" can replace the perception of "value for money" that now drives our food system, says food policy expert Tim Lang.[28] Pay the Price is one European group educating consumers to tolerate higher prices for sustainable food. The project began as a Facebook page, but Pay the Price gained so much support that it is now a think-tank examining the international food industry and working to get hidden costs included in retail rates.[29] Environmentalist Robert Kennedy Jr. is optimistic, and says "Americans know good food when they taste it, and choose sustainability even when it costs more."[30]

Limit your seafood and dairy intake, too, and find good sources.

Seafood and dairy also need moderation. When moving meat to the side of the plate, don't just replace it with more cheese or fish. Excessive dairy or seafood have their own ways of adding to environmental and health problems. Start with smaller amounts. At seafood restaurants, share a salmon or shrimp meal with a friend or family member. You'll be unlikely to go hungry, given standard portion sizes, and you can order a few vegetables on the side.

When shopping for fish, look for local species native to your part of the world, so they don't need to be airfreighted to your table. Eat more wild fish than farmed ones. Move away from carnivorous species and toward smaller fish lower on the food chain. This takes commitment, since the most popular fish foods in North America include salmon, tuna, and cod, all of which eat a lot of small fish to get big. Try eating more sardines, mackerel, herring, and anchovies. Those fish feed solely on vegetable matter, using less of the Earth's resources, to get to edible size.[31]

Look for eco-labels showing that environmental organizations approve of the fish you're buying. Eco-labels are an evolving science.[32] One comprehensive analysis of seafood eco-labels[33] gave high environmental ratings to the US National Organic Standard, the Soil Association, the Salmon Aquaculture Dialogue, and some others. There are many labels from organizations that additionally educate and work for policy change. SeaChoice is one, backed by groups including the David Suzuki Foundation and the Sierra Club, in collaboration with the Seafood Watch program at the Monterey Bay Aquarium.[34]

Seek out retailers who care. One Toronto seafood store, Hooked, sells only species that are not endangered and that have been caught with limited impact on the environment and other marine life.[35]

Farmed seafood, grown using aquaculture methods, can in some cases be a sustainable option. However, farmed shrimp and prawns are often ecologically detrimental because some are grown in coastal ponds, such as those in Southeast Asia, which were created through destruction of mangroves and wetland habitats. As well, environmental organizations advise caution on seafood from "open net" farms. These farms are adjacent to coastlines, where ocean water sloshes in and out, allowing fish-farm chemicals and biological waste to diffuse into the open waters and potentially contaminate wild species. Unfortunately, aquaculture operations often focus on growing salmon and other carnivorous fish, which puts pressure on wild stocks of smaller fish that end up as feed.

Consumers are concerned. According to a recent World Wildlife Fund Canada study, more than 90% of Canadians feel it is important that their fish and other seafood come from sustainable stocks that have not been overfished. But only 8% felt they have adequate information on the source of their seafood.[36]

Dairy products also require moderation if we're going to consume them sustainably. That means eating smaller amounts that come from sources that produce the milk, eggs, and cheese consistent with local ecosystems. Buying dairy products that are certified organic is a good start, as is getting to know local producers. Eggs that have been produced in various ways are often available, including organic and free-range.[37] For details, contact a local humane society or natural foods retailer.

Eat, drink, and be merry.[38]

That may sound self-explanatory. But you'll be more merry if you remember a few points of compassion for others and for yourself.

First, there's no need to stop eating meat or to give up anything. Vegetarians deserve our respect, but we can partake of animal products conscientiously by significantly lowering our meat intake and buying from the best kinds of farms.

Second, no one is asking poor or undernourished people to decrease their intake. A movement to eat less meat is aimed at people who buy animal products regularly and who have other options. If you're a regular meat-eater, you qualify.

Third, we can help put an end to the polarized debate between meat-eaters and vegetarians. Act cooperatively and work with everyone, no matter what they eat. Whether you consider yourself a meat-eater, a vegetarian, or something in between, you can take a nuanced view of dietary preferences rather than worry about labels. As you alter your own eating habits, do so in ways that respect family and housemates. It's a nice aspect of the "eat less meat" approach that it is easy to accommodate others while you make changes for yourself. Eventually, they may join in your quest to moderate the meat binge.

We Can Be Healthier by Eating Less Meat

How do you stay healthy if you're eating less meat? It's certainly the case that people who are undernourished get healthier if they eat some meat or other animal products. But most of us are not in that category, and would be much better off with less. And for humans as a whole, we don't need any meat to survive and thrive, as long as we get a wide range of plant-based foods. We're not primarily carnivores, but highly adaptable omnivores.

Low-meat diets that are well-rounded can provide adequate protein, iron, and other nutrients. You can also get all you need for physical well-being from vegetarian diets and even from vegan ones, which include no animal products.[39] Whether you eat meat is not the deciding factor in whether your diet is a healthy one. You can eat well with few animal products if you include a variety of vegetables, legumes, grains, and fruits, and minimize highly processed foods loaded with salt, fat, and sugar.

Protein is the issue on most people's minds when considering a reduced-meat diet. Vegetarians are constantly asked by friends and family how they get enough, but sufficient good-quality protein is easily obtainable on low-meat or no-meat diets. The meat industry has worked hard to make "protein" seem synonymous with meat,[40] but many other foods contain this macronutrient in good quantity and quality. Nutritional science shows it's not difficult to get ample protein from modest servings of beans, lentils, nuts, and even foods we don't consider sources of protein such as whole-wheat bread, potatoes, and grains.

Most of us appear to take in much more protein than we need or is good for us. According to scientists David and Marcia Pimentel, average Americans eat twice the recommended daily allowance of protein per adult per day.[41] That's backed up by the Food and Agriculture Organization, which says a safe level of protein consumption for average adults is 58 grams a day (about 2 ounces), while average protein consumption in the United States from 2003–2005 was 116 grams (about 4 ounces) per person per day.[42] Most American protein intake is from animal products, and that's part of the problem because these also contain significant amounts of cholesterol and fat. Meanwhile, excesses of protein cause their own health problems. For example, too much can promote calcium excretion, which may make us more vulnerable to osteoporosis.[43]

Most recommendations say Americans can get all the protein they need while eating less meat. The US Department of Agriculture food pyramid recommends 2 or 3 protein servings a day, and its graphic representation of a healthy meal shows proteins taking up less than one quarter of the plate.[44] But your protein doesn't need to come from animal sources, so you don't need any, or many, animal products if you eat a few baked beans, or some whole-wheat toast with peanut butter, or morning oatmeal with soymilk, or other protein-containing plant foods. Canada's Food Guide, another tool for healthy and balanced meals, underscores the need for protein but points out that there are many sources. "Have meat alternatives such as beans, lentils and tofu often," says the national guide, which also recommends dry roasted nuts and seeds (without extra oil and salt) as part of the "meat and alternatives" group.[45]

How Much Protein Do You Need?

We all require protein in our diets. But most of us take in more than is necessary or even healthy, according to a growing list of nutrition experts and studies, including those cited in this chapter. They remind us that plant-based meals can provide good-quality protein and that, as long as you eat a wide range of wholesome foods, you can get plenty of this nutrient with little in the way of meat, dairy products, or fish.

"Many people mistakenly believe a common meat myth that you can't get a healthy amount of protein from a vegetarian diet. Not true," states Dawn Jackson Blatner, dietitian and author of *The Flexitarian Diet* who counsels people to eat well with a minimum of animal products. She gives an example of a daily meal plan: For breakfast: cereal with soy milk topped with nuts and berries. For lunch: 1½ cups of black bean soup with a salad and whole-grain roll. For a snack: an apple with peanut butter. For dinner: a barbequed veggie burger with sweet potato fries. Overall, that meal plan gives you 60 grams (about 2 ounces) of protein for the day, which Ms. Blatner says is enough for most people.

Nutritionists emphasize that there's no simple answer to how much protein or how many daily calories people need, since optimal amounts depend on age, weight, level of exercise, state of health, and other factors. And there are individuals who need extra protein. But according to dietary authority Marion Nestle: "Even if you are a vegan and eat no animal products at all, you almost certainly get more than enough protein from the grains, beans, and vegetables you eat."

Sources: Dawn Jackson Blatner, *The Flexitarian Diet: The Mostly Vegetarian Way to Lose Weight, Be Healthier, Prevent Disease, and Add Years to Your Life.* NY: McGraw Hill, 2009, p. 18; Marion Nestle, *What to Eat: An Aisle-by-Aisle Guide to Savvy Food Choices and Good Eating.* NY: North Point Press, 2006, p. 143.

People wanting to cut back on meat are also concerned whether a low-meat diet will give them high-quality or complete protein. To that, many nutritionists say that plant protein is as good as animal protein for human health as long as you're eating a wide variety of foods. While animal foods are a convenient source of complete protein, plant protein is more than adequate. As Vesanto Melina and Brenda Davis, authors of *Becoming Vegetarian* write: "We now recognize that a varied diet of plant foods suits human protein needs very well."[46]

To get satisfactory nutrients on a low-meat diet, eat lots of green and colored vegetables, whole grains and breads, fruit, beans, and other legumes. If the latter sound odd to you, think of them in familiar forms as pea soup, pinto or black beans in tortillas, and Indian lentils, and remember that many well-known dishes, such as vegetarian chili and minestrone soup, contain legumes.

We've Already Started This Project

Eating less meat is an extension of some of the dietary changes many of us have already made in trying to eat local, organic, healthy food. Some people are gradually eating less meat, as illustrated by new phrases in our lexicon such as "part-time vegetarian," "weekday vegetarian," and "flexitarian" for people who eat meat but don't identify as primarily carnivorous. More and more people are involved, including Free the Children cofounders Craig and Marc Kielburger. Famous for rallying tens of thousands of young people at inspirational events for social change, the brothers have written about their struggle to give up steak and shrimp. In a recent article, they show they're limiting their meat and calling themselves "flexivores."[47]

Eating less meat also builds on other non-food environmental actions many of us have taken. You're probably recycling, riding your bike, and opting for more public transit rather than driving everywhere. Eating less meat is the next big step. Engaging in this project is also consistent with the values we already try to live. Supporting sustainable and compassionate production fits with who we are and who we want to be.

You won't be alone in cutting your meat consumption; you'll be joining a sweeping movement already populated by celebrities and scientists. You'll be joining politician, scientist, and climate-change expert Al Gore, who has decreased his meat consumption. You'll be in company with musician and activist Paul McCartney, a spokesperson for England's version of Meatless Monday. You'll be joining food writers Michael Pollan and Mark Bittman, who advise people to lower their consumption of animal products. You'll be in the same boat as environmentalist Graham Hill, who declares himself a weekday vegetarian. You'll be in the same club as Annie Somerville of the restaurant Greens. You'll be part of a worldwide movement.

Citizen action on a large scale is a modern phenomenon that provides an optimistic basis for this project and demonstrates the power of individual choice. People and their actions have transformed the world and can transform our food systems. As documented by Paul Hawken in *Blessed Unrest*,[48] citizen action can change the world.

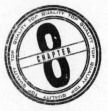

FOOD POLICY CAN ENSURE
SUSTAINABLE PRODUCTION

Taxes Could Be on the Table

Taxes on meat are a policy option that Hans Schreier has been advocating for years. "I used to suggest the idea at international conferences, and people would laugh," said the professor in an interview.[1] But the time has come to consider even controversial ideas for addressing the ecological and health problems of livestock and meat.

Taxing sausages and prime rib may sound far-fetched, but it's worth a debate. Dr. Schreier, an international water expert at the University of British Columbia's Institute for Resources, Environment and Sustainability, has recommended strong government policy to address the global crises of water shortages and pollution.[2] He has also frankly suggested retail taxes on meat,[3] and in this he is not alone. "Consumption taxes should be imposed on animal food," say Swedish scientists Stefan Wirsenius and Fredrik Hedenus,[4] to discourage heavy intake of meals that use more than their share of resources and produce more than their share of gas emissions. Taxes could be based on the level of emissions for each food type, which would raise retail prices on chicken wings and pork chops, and even more on beef.

There's nothing radical about taxing foods and drugs that, in excess, can harm health and the environment. European countries tax a range of processed meal items, and they are considering further action.[5] In North America, some jurisdictions tax soft drinks, and more are considering it.[6] We also apply heavy taxes to alcohol and cigarettes. Denmark has taken the leap of applying levies to fatty foods, including meat, by imposing a "fat tax" on lipid-heavy products, thus increasing retail prices of foods like hamburgers and butter.[7] But that's Europe, where citizens historically have been more likely to accept personal limits for the common good. Scientists and commentators in the United States and Canada are more reluctant to advocate retail price increases, though a few have done so.[8]

Nevertheless, taxes on animal products are worth putting on the table for discussion, especially given that such fiscal measures can shift consumption in more ecological directions. "Having been banished to the bottom of the list of policy options to address unhealthy eating for years, food taxes are now gaining the favour of European policy makers," observes UK public health specialist Dr. Corinna Hawkes.[9] Though predicting consumer response isn't easy, taxes can influence consumption in pro-social directions. A report from the Organization for Economic Cooperation and Development (OECD) showed that taxes in various countries have helped limit car emissions, household energy consumption, water use, and household waste.[10] It only works if taxes are substantial enough to really play a role in consumers' calculations. Other researchers have noted that taxing bad food and subsidizing good food can encourage healthier choices.[11] In Ireland, higher taxes on soft drinks led to less consumption, and in Denmark, subsidizing fruits, vegetables, and specific nutrients led people to consume more of them.

So taxes would probably lower consumption — though whether a little or a lot would depend on factors such as how essential consumers believe meat to be, and what alternatives they're ready and able to purchase, as discussed in Chapter 6. There are growing numbers of consumers who do not consider meat a must-have daily food, and public education could further popularize that perception. Meat taxes could also play a role in acclimatizing consumers to paying more. Eventually, expectations would shift, and higher prices wouldn't look so out of line. This isn't a wild idea, since there is evidence that some consumers are becoming willing to pay more for better meat, as outlined in Chapter 7.[12]

We can expect controversy. In New Zealand in 2003, officials proposed a livestock "flatulence tax" to fund research on reducing emissions for compliance with the Kyoto Protocol on climate change. But the initiative was opposed by agricultural groups.[13] Since then, New Zealand, where up to half of greenhouse gas emissions come from farm animals, has been back at the drawing board for alternative strategies to reduce livestock emissions and pollution.

If people aren't too shocked by the idea of a meat tax, we could take the discussion a step further and consider a wartime strategy. That's rationing. A few courageous analysts have raised the topic, suggesting that our governments explicitly limit the amount of meat that any individual can purchase in a week or a month. It was standard practice during World War II in some countries, but today we're accustomed to having whatever we can buy.

If we're serious about tackling climate change, the effort "will indeed entail going onto some kind of 'war footing,'" in the view of UK sustainability commentator Jonathon Porritt.[14] The long-serving former chair of his country's Sustainable Development Commission, Mr. Porritt believes there are two human behaviors "that simply cannot be squared with any reasonable scenario of a genuinely sustainable future for humankind." One is frequent air travel, and "the second is the continuing growth in demand for meat consumption,"[15] which, he says, is impossible to maintain even at current levels, let alone at the higher levels projected. His suggestion is PMQs, or Personal Meat Quotas. It's rationing, pure and simple.

One rationale for rationing is fairness. If we simply tax meat, it could become food for the wealthy, or the policy could disproportionately (and regressively) burden the poor, though authorities could come up with strategies to assist low-income consumers. But under a rationing system, every citizen would be accorded a standard quota. Rationing would also allow officials to coax citizens from heavy to moderate meat consumption, through a gradual decrease in rations.

There's little chance rationing would be publicly accepted today, unless citizens widely believed that we had an emergency. That was the case in World War II Britain, where tens of millions of citizens lived with the Ministry of Food's strict rationing on many items, including meat and dairy products. While there was occasional grumbling, most people accepted or even welcomed the sacrifices, believing that the war was just and that the government needed to manage food supplies.[16] According to the late historian Tony Judt, "the British proved remarkably tolerant of their deprivations — in part because of a belief that these were, at least, shared fairly across the community."[17] But there was a war on, and the war was considered necessary, given the terrible threat. Today the imperative is less clear. Yet many believe we are in an undeclared war for the health of the planet and survival of humanity, and so far it's not clear we'll win. Perhaps we can take some lessons from the wartime Ministry of Food.[18]

Extraordinary public officials would be needed to promote such initiatives — even taxes, let alone stronger measures. "Scary prospect for our politicians?" asks Mr. Porritt. "Of course. For people who see cheap meat as part of their latter-day birthright, such a proposal is a total anathema."[19] So let's see if we can find some extraordinary public officials.

Meat Policy Should Be Central to Food Policy

The meat problem presents a prototype of dilemmas found throughout the food system: pollution and degradation of land and water; excessive corporate concentration; loss of local control and rural communities; overprocessing of foods for more convenience, but less health; a retreat from simple and naturally grown sustenance; and aggressive marketing of so-called value-added foods rather than fresh vegetables, grains, and fruits. These are some of the realities that inspire people to roll up their sleeves and work for better food policy. Meanwhile, there's probably no category of food that causes more of those problems than animal products, and there's no food sector with a more pressing need for visionary planning. But the topic continues to be downplayed, and in discussions of food policy, meat remains the fleshy elephant in the room. The need for governments to address the problems of livestock and meat was clearly pronounced in 2006 by the authors of *Livestock's Long Shadow*:

> Livestock-environment interactions are not easily understood. They are broad and complex, and many of the impacts are indirect and not obvious, so it is easy to underestimate livestock's impact on land and land use, climate change, water and biodiversity. ...A policy framework conducive to more environmentally benign practices simply does not exist in many cases, or is rudimentary at best. ...For the most part, livestock's impact on the environment does not receive an appropriate policy response, even though the technical means to do so exist.[20]

Meat can be seen as a barometer for whether food policy can succeed, says Tim Lang, professor at City University in London and head of the Centre for Food Policy. "Because of its deep impact, meat is a test case for how and whether policymakers align the food system with sustainability goals," he and his colleagues have written. "To reshape meat production and consumption, and to bring them in line with the Earth's capacities, is a microcosm of challenges facing both the food system and the way humans live and relate with the biosphere."[21]

Food policy is becoming a hot topic as governments, researchers, and citizen groups realize the need to feed people well without wrecking the planet or public health. Everyone recognizes there are problems with food production, distribution, and consumption, though they may not agree on solutions. Nevertheless, when people talk about food policy, they're talking about overarching legislative frameworks and practices for making sufficient good food for billions of people, while supporting ecosystems and community well-being.

The idea that countries need food policy is catching on internationally, due in part to pioneers like Dr. Lang. In Canada, the idea has inspired proposals by major political parties.[22] Agriculture and policy organizations have published reports on the topic.[23] The idea sparked The People's Food Policy Project of the non-governmental organization Food Secure Canada, which gathered ideas from citizens and published the report, "Resetting the Table," calling for national policies to provide food for all, support farmers and fishers, ensure that food is produced within ecological limits, and encourage healthy consumption.[24]

Food policy doesn't really even exist in many industrialized countries. That's the view of Environmental Studies Professor Rod MacRae of York University in Toronto, who has studied this issue for years. Dr. MacRae has written an ambitious overview of what's needed, outlining the kinds of principles, values, and goals that could drive healthy food systems.[25] Canada has agricultural policies, trade policies, and nutrition policies but no coordinated, well-articulated food policies. What's needed is a "joined-up" framework that would be "comprehensive" and "system-wide" to oversee food production and consumption and steer them in directions consistent with economic goals as well as environmental health.[26] Agriculture is rarely publicly debated by elected officials, except for dramatic events concerning food safety or political tugs-of-war over commodity marketing. By and large, decisions are being made at bureaucratic levels. "But food," he says, "is too important for that."[27]

It's not that food systems don't exist, or we would never find anything at the grocery store. It's that no one seems to be in charge with a long-term vision for agriculture and food based on what Dr. Lang calls "ecological public health."[28] I'm reminded of a conversation I had with an industrial food lobbyist. In a candid moment, he described meetings between agriculture executives and government officials wanting to encourage intensive meat production. "And it felt like there was nobody there representing the public interest."

Whether or not a society deliberately shapes food policy, it nevertheless gets shaped. Officially, rules for business are drawn up by international trade agreements and a network of governments. But the system is such that agribusiness helps write the food rules,[29] so policy is strongly influenced by corporate stakeholders or, in the case of meat, steakholders. Food policy could be organized more deliberately, with the public interest front and center.

Food policy that is comprehensive would help shift agriculture toward fewer chemicals, lower energy inputs, and less environmental damage. This is a complicated business, as Dr. MacRae has studied in relation to organic agriculture. Even when conventional farmers want to transition to chemical-free agriculture, governments aren't always in positions to help, for reasons ranging from logistics to politics. Officials can have trouble appreciating organic farming. It's a complete system rather than a series of discrete technologies and practices; organic farming seems small and marginal, and its environmental benefits are not always understood.[30] Those benefits are well documented, including in a 2011 study from pioneer organic organization the Rodale Institute, based in Pennsylvania. A 30-year comparison between organic farming and the conventional chemical kind showed that, after an initial transition period, organic methods produced as much yield, performed better in drought years, built up the soil rather than depleting it of plant matter, used less energy, and were even more profitable.[31] Yet governments aren't always flexible enough to recognize and bolster environmentally superior ways of doing things.

Food policy needs to think big in other ways if it is to resist being pigeonholed in one government department and one artificial policy silo. Better to work across ministries and departments, bringing together relevant people and matters — even though they're usually considered distinct — including agriculture, industry, nutrition, and trade.

Food policymakers need to think expansively about food safety. It's often in the news, as the media report on *E. coli* contaminations of grocery items or diseases sweeping animal herds. We're so accustomed to large numbers that we're desensitized, but in Iowa in 2010, hundreds of millions of eggs were recalled in more than ten states after a salmonella outbreak related to intensive farms.[32] Listeriosis became a public health issue in 2008 when some Canadian consumers got the disease from a bacterial infection "linked to ready-to-eat meats" from an Ontario meat processing plant.[33] The outbreak took 22 lives and made 35 other people seriously ill. An investigator made more than 50 important recommendations to minimize the likelihood of future such events.[34] In both these cases, detailed examinations were conducted to find out which factories were responsible and, in some cases, even which production lines.

But food safety is bigger than the front page, and contaminations aren't ultimately the fault of one production line. At some point, we need to examine industrial food production itself. "Each step in the modern food chain increases the chance of food contamination," says the Canadian government.[35] We need to dig deeper and question the underlying production paradigms and consumer expectations that may be larger threats to food safety.

Food policy needs to expand its vision outside the technological box. No farmer wants to be without appropriate technology, even if it's just electric fencing, basic farm equipment, or a laptop. But with a limited future for cheap oil, and growing evidence that small-scale farming can be highly productive, we'll need to encourage farms that don't rely on multi-million dollar equipment, fertilizers, and chemicals. High-tech approaches to our problems can seem attractive when they offer quick fixes that don't require us to change personal habits or production systems. It's tempting to think we can keep eating hamburgers daily if we take anti-cholesterol drugs. It's tempting to think we can keep producing billions of food animals if we use technologies like vaccines to decrease their methane output.[36] These might seem logical within a narrow framework of reductionist science. But for the long term, we'll want to consider an alternative strategy — to produce animals in lower densities and consume the products of those animals in lower amounts, appropriate to ecosystems and to health.

To think beyond technology, we need to question approaches such as genetic modification of food, also called genetic engineering, which sound good when biotechnology companies describe them. Biotech representatives contend that their products confer desirable characteristics and improve food yields,[37] and at least two genetically modified livestock species are awaiting government endorsement. Scientists at the University of Guelph are seeking approvals to move along on their lab-engineered pig that purportedly excretes less phosphorus.[38] Another company is seeking permission to market an engineered salmon that grows faster than the usual.[39] But critics of genetic engineering say there's little evidence of upsides, lots of unknown consequences and potential environmental downsides, and the hard-to-dispute consequence that genetic engineering concentrates power in the hands of the few corporations that are granted legal patents over the organisms and their offspring.[40]

Food policy needs to take a step that may seem like fantasy in city-centric life: It needs to help people move back to the farm. Sustainable farming requires more labor than does conventional farming, and it will need revitalized, repopulated countrysides. Along with that, rural regions will need a re-emergence of local infrastructure such as fruit canning and fish processing of the sort that, in many of our regions, are long gone.

How 'ya gonna keep 'em down on the farm...after they've seen the big city? That's what a popular song asked during World War I,[41] and indeed millions deliberately choose urban life. But there remain many who would love to move to an acreage if small-scale food production offered a decent living. As a result, initiatives are arising to help young people realize that dream and to encourage more families to consider farm life and help repopulate countrysides. There are moves for modern homestead acts. I recently saw an e-discussion of a proposed Beginning Farmer and Rancher Opportunity Act.[42] In Ontario, there is an organization called FarmStart to help people pursue agricultural careers, and there are other programs and organizations working toward similar goals.[43] The number of farms is actually increasing in some parts of the United States, notes leading environmentalist Bill McKibben, as serious people begin to realize the role of small-scale agriculture in sustainability.[44] People may have asked 90 years ago "how 'ya gonna keep 'em down on the farm?" but when singer Elton John released "Goodbye Yellow Brick Road" more than 50 years later, telling of a man who abandoned city life to return to his plow and his family farm, the album sold more than 30 million copies. Food policy can sell itself, too, and shape smarter systems for livestock and meat production.

Policy Can Encourage Healthy Consumption

Years ago when friends came for dinner, I always served meat. Familiar cuts were affordable, and I knew how to cook beef, chicken, and pork. Little did I know my personal choices were shaped to make meat low-priced, convenient, and socially expected. In earlier chapters, I discussed how sanctioned practices can shape production and consumption. The complexity of policy, and of food systems, can make it seem impossible to challenge the meat binge. It can make us feel that we have little practical alternative but to rely on chicken and steak. But if policy can cause problems, it can solve them, too, and complexity presents the opportunity for numerous points of intervention.

Policy tools that can foster real change come in many shapes and sizes. Some are regulatory and others economic, though the two are not entirely distinct and can converge on the same aims. Regulatory or "command and control" approaches often set standards or limits. In terms of meat production, industries could be required to employ certain pollution control technologies, and companies that don't comply would be fined. Economic approaches could include imposing fees or taxes on polluters for their discharges. Or, an economic solution via a different route would be offering financial rewards for sustainable practices. Each approach has advantages and disadvantages and is appropriate to different situations. There are, of course, many other tools that could be used. Public information campaigns are an obvious choice for this topic because it affects practically everyone. One memorable way of viewing policy options is, in the words of Professor Rod MacRae, "carrots, sticks, or sermons" — incentives, disincentives, or education.[45] Any or all of these can be used to reach sustainability goals.

Policy options can also be seen as targeting either consumption or production — demand or supply — though these aren't completely separate either, since the two affect and complement each other. On the supply side, governments can increase prices of resource inputs to meat production (or stop subsidizing those inputs), disallow certain chemicals in feeds and factory farms, and limit corporate concentration in the industry. On the demand side, governments could educate consumers to eat differently, or increase prices through taxation. Because changes to supply affect demand, there are many ways we could help consumers eat differently by requiring production systems to make less and make it better. This could be done through combinations of legislation, regulation, and commitment to enforcement. Governments can take steps to stop fueling the binge.

If policymakers decide to stick to a gentle approach for adjusting consumption, public education programs could be organized in partnership with health agencies and non-governmental organizations already working on this project—from the New York-based Sustainable Table, to the California-based EarthSave, to the Physicians' Committee for Responsible Medicine in Washington.[46] Policymakers could use existing channels to engage with various demographics, using media both new and old.

But public information may not suffice. "Education alone is no match for marketing dollars," says food writer Mark Bittman.[47] He's referring mostly to promotion of processed foods, but also states flatly that we eat too many animal products for the environment or health. Fast food, animal products, and highly processed snacks are heavily marketed, he says, with the US fast-food industry spending billions in advertising—while offices for nutrition policy and promotion have budgets that are a fraction of that.[48] Advertising is a powerful tool for affecting consumer choice, and governments could consider judicious limits to the marketing of meat and dairy. Our governments already disallow ads they judge to be unfair or deceptive, and they limit advertising for products such as cigarettes and alcohol that are harmful if overused or misused. We know that advertising can fuel excessive consumption so, as another potential approach, we could consider the opposite: advertising healthy eating.

Policy Can Improve Livestock Production

It is possible to raise livestock with a soft ecological footprint and with respect for animals and nature. That's what's being done in thousands of agricultural operations around North America, where dedicated farmers are applying environmental, ethical, health, and social standards to the natural rearing of animals for food. For example, the Niman Ranch in northern California started almost 40 years ago raising cattle traditionally and has expanded to include more than 650 American farmers and ranchers who produce beef, pork, and lamb humanely and with

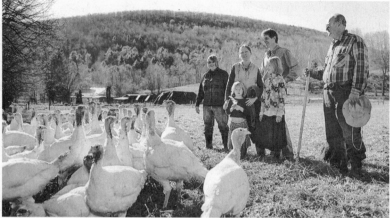

The Hayes family on their Sap Bush Hollow Farm in upstate New York.
L to R: (rear) Adele Hayes, Shannon Hayes and her husband Bob Hooper,
Jim Hayes. Front: Shannon and Bob's girls, Ula and Saoirse.

no hormones or antibiotics.[49] The Good Shepherd Poultry operation
based in Tampa, Kansas, raises "historically authentic heritage" birds
that are free-range, vegetarian fed, and antibiotic-free.[50] Owner Frank
Reese Jr. says he also goes one step further, by breeding his own heritage
birds "without ever buying genetics from the factory farm system."[51]
Demonstrating that you can make a fair amount of food this way, Good
Shepherd works with nearby farms to produce and sell 1,500 chickens
each week and about 8,000 turkeys a year.[52]

Sap Bush Hollow Farm near Albany in upstate New York is another
example of sustainability, where Jim and Adele Hayes, along with their
daughter Shannon and her family, raise grassfed lamb and beef, plus
pastured pork and poultry. Committed to chemical-free agriculture,
these farmers range a few dozen cattle and pigs, about a thousand
chickens, and some turkeys and laying hens. They concede their meat
may appear more expensive than conventional cuts. "But price is only
a factor if people don't understand the true costs of their food," says
Adele. "Grassfed and pastured meats do not cost more, people are just
paying for the other meat through their taxes/farm subsidies so that it
looks cheaper in the grocery store."[53]

The Hayes family is engaged in what they do. Shannon and her father Jim have extensive formal training in agriculture and animal science, and the whole family educates the public by writing, giving speeches at local and national conferences, and consulting to farm groups. Shannon's books include *The Grassfed Gourmet Cookbook*[54] which outlines the why and how of preparing meat meals that are good for health and the Earth. Members of the Hayes clan run a "grassfed intern" program to teach people the business of ecological meat production. They demonstrate that it can be done, as do approximately 10,000 other sustainable producers of animal products in the United States.[55]

But these kinds of farms turn out a minority of our meat, dairy, and eggs. With most of our animal foods emerging from factories, transforming livestock systems from animal warehouses and assembly lines to natural farms like Sap Bush Hollow won't be easy. And there's no obvious path for government policymakers to follow to get from here to there. Yet policy needs to target the supply side, employing laws and regulations to limit the most problematic of factory farm practices and support cleaner and kinder production. A lot of the approaches come down to supporting sustainable production, but sometimes it involves just not getting in the way. I've had livestock ranchers tell me that they don't need government to do much for them — if it would just stop policies and practices that advantage the factory-farm competition.

There is a wide range of available strategies to make livestock and meat better both for now and for the future. Central to it all is a need for governments to re-examine their assumptions about what constitutes desirable livestock and meat production. Governments can improve decision-making about where livestock operations are allowed to locate — at the very least enforce restrictions on CAFOs in environmentally sensitive regions. Authorities can reform tax structures and rethink public policies that affect the pricing of resources like water and commodities like corn. They can reward livestock producers for practices that limit greenhouse gases.[56] Rewards would encourage farmers to adopt more sustainable practices we already know would be helpful: reducing emissions from ruminant burps and manure; avoiding feed from deforested regions; preserving and building carbon in crop and grazing lands; and otherwise improving land management. Policy can set standards for producers on pesticide use, water quality, ammonia emissions, and greenhouse gas release.[57]

Some producers are beginning to make livestock systems more sustainable. Manitoba pork companies are aiming to decrease greenhouse gases and limit water contamination, especially during spring runoff.[58] One major US-based meat processor says it is working on decreasing its water use, analyzing and lowering its gas emissions, and figuring out ways to minimize its pollution.[59] But dramatic improvements, in any region and by any company, may not be achieved voluntarily. Producers have large investments in current systems, and are not always certain that alternative methods will allow them to meet their financial objectives. In current business systems, companies understandably hesitate to take expensive steps for sustainability that aren't required either by consumer demand or by law — especially if their competitors aren't taking the same steps. Besides, they have their hands full dealing with other pressures, such as increasing feed and energy prices and international competition.

If we want different livestock systems, we'll need different public policy. A good place to start would be requiring lower densities — by capping animal numbers per unit of land — that will better integrate livestock into ecosystems.[60] De-intensify, says Dr. MacRae, and you will contribute to solving other environmental, social, health, and ethical problems in food production.

Any sustainable rancher or farmer knows they need to keep animals in densities low enough to suit local ecosystems. They can't graze and pasture animals in ways that degrade the land. But that doesn't mean good livestock operations are necessarily small. Some have only a few dozen acres, but in the rangy interior of British Columbia, Empire Valley Ranch produces sustainable beef on more than 300,000 acres — more than half the size of Rhode Island. On this awesome piece of land, which was leased from the government, Joyce Holmes and her family run 500 mother cattle, 25 Angus bulls, plus calves, and none of them are given chemicals, hormones, or antibiotics. As another rancher told me, good livestock ranching can come in packages large or small. There's no magic formula for size. Density is a more important feature than size.

Whatever the scale of livestock operations, policy can ensure that operators pay the full costs of production. Today, there are costs in intensive meat-making that don't get properly shouldered by producers. In the United States, these have included supports to keep prices low for livestock feed and lax enforcement on cleanup and manure management.[61] You don't need to be an economist to agree that it's not wise to allow businesses to offload such costs onto taxpayers and society, creating what economists call "externalities." Many observers agree that agricultural externalities need to be internalized, and rightly paid for by producers.[62] Industry analysts have plenty of ideas on how to achieve that.[63] What's needed is political will — with a dose of creativity and courage.

Support sustainable producers and stop supporting unsustainable ones. That's what public policy could do, but programs today tend to favor industrial producers. Large corporations benefit disproportionately from agricultural support money, and livestock producers are directly or indirectly among the top recipients.[64] Environmental writer Bill McKibben suggests that 60% of supports go to the largest 10% of US farms.[65] However, agricultural economist Dr. Gary Williams cautions against demonizing corporate farms for benefiting from government subsidies. Many of these large farms really are family farms, he told a recent Harvard University forum. "Some of them are very big because they've been very successful. But that doesn't mean they're the problem."[66] It comes down to a need for systematic policy — for deliberate decisions to encourage agriculture in a range of sizes if it is to be sustainable, safe, and healthy.

Subsidies are a strong presence in industrial agriculture; they make up almost a third of farm income in Western countries.[67] Yet they remain a multi-billion dollar controversy, and feedstuffs for livestock are at the heart of the issue.[68] US farm policy has used a range of incentive measures to encourage massive production of corn and soy. This has allowed commodity producers to churn out billions of bushels of corn each year and sell it as feed to livestock corporations at prices below the cost of production. The system amounts to a subsidy to grain-fed beef, chicken, and pork. It's been itemized by researchers Elanor Starmer and

Timothy Wise of Tufts University, who calculated that industrial live-stock firms saved almost $4 billion each year between 1997 and 2005 by purchasing subsidized feedstuffs, saving 5–15% on their operating costs.[69] This situation is changing as corn and other prices rise based on surging demand for ethanol and alternative uses. But crop subsidies have been a major factor in the rise and market dominance of intensive livestock.[70]

In the United States, such subsidies are codified under the contro-versial Farm Bill, which is the subject of intensive negotiations and lobbying. The Farm Bill "is a tremendous opportunity," says analyst Daniel Imhoff. "Used correctly, it can incentivize an agriculture and food system that remedies rather than perpetuates many of today's problems."[71] For that to happen, officials will need to use legislation to assist the best kinds of food producers.

Governments' supports to industrial agriculture also come in other forms. Tax policies frequently reward big and punish small, in some jurisdictions by allowing animal facilities to be taxed as farms rather than the industries that some consider them to be. "Factory farms are taxed at the same rate as other farms, yet they use a higher propor-tion of community services," says the Citizens' Guide to Confronting a Factory Farm.[72] Intensive farms use large amounts of water and cause heavy truck traffic to haul feed and transport animals, stirring up dust and damaging roads. Additionally, tax laws can burden small-scale farms. In Ontario, even if a family spends most of its time producing meat, milk, vegetables, grain, and other foods for themselves and oth-ers, they may not officially be regarded as farming, says rural writer Thomas Pawlick. They cannot claim the lower farm rate of property tax unless they sell thousands of dollars of food each year. "They are in-stead taxed at the same rate as a wealthy urban resident who purchases a lakeside cottage to use for summer holidays, and makes no effort to do anything on the property other than sunbathe."[73]

Supports to industrial agriculture sometimes come in the form of barriers to small-scale production. Government meat inspection is one example. In British Columbia, it's been a sore point since the Province moved to implement new rules that no meat be sold for human consumption unless it has been fully inspected and slaughtered in a provincially or federally licensed facility. The rules would make it illegal for many small rural producers to sell their meat locally, even though their practices might be sustainable, healthy, and humane.[74] It's not that such policies deliberately set out to undermine local farmers, but when systems are designed for large processors, small ones can find it too difficult or too costly to comply.

Governments don't like to admit that their policies favor some producers over others, says Dr. MacRae. Agricultural subsidies in Canada run into the billions of dollars a year, but still are relatively modest compared with those in the United States. But Canadian support programs are "clearly focused on the 20% of highest-volume producers."[75] If farms aren't generating substantial sales, they're not of much interest to government, which gets nudged by agribusiness not to waste time and money on smallholders they deride as hobby farmers.[76]

Pork provides an example of policies that advantage big meat, or, in this case, big pig. Federal and provincial governments have offered numerous kinds of financial help to factory hog farms. In Manitoba, hog producers have benefitted from public money for special projects, labor subsidies to bring in foreign workers, and tax dollars to help build roads and other infrastructure.[77] Factory farms have received millions of dollars in public loans. When meat companies have shown interest in expanding on the Prairies, provinces have competed for the business.[78]

One example of policies favorable to mass-scale producers involves the messy topic of manure. Environmentalists claim that CAFOs and ILOs get cut a lot of slack from governments on waste management, not only through lack of strict enforcement on regulations but even through direct assistance with waste disposal.[79] In the United States, tens of millions of taxpayers' dollars each year are directed to build and fortify manure lagoons on CAFOs and corporate feedlots, under the Environmental Quality Incentives Program or EQIP.[80] "Although the reduction of harm caused by CAFOs is desirable, EQIP payments raise legitimate questions about whether the public should underwrite CAFOs in this way," points out Dr. Doug Gurian-Sherman, of the Union of Concerned

Scientists, in his important 2008 analysis of environmental challenges in meat production.[81] Many jurisdictions pay CAFOs to comply with manure-management legislation. In Canada, the Ontario government provided millions of dollars in 2005 alone to help large livestock operations handle waste.[82] This might sound socially beneficial, but meanwhile, others go to the trouble and expense of integrating manure into crop production.

It raises the question of how much governments should help producers comply with environmental standards. Manitoba has a ban on winter spreading of manure. Another phase of this ban is scheduled to take effect in November 2013, and some livestock producers say they need financial assistance.[83] These kinds of situations present opportunities and potential levers for authorities to assist producers only when they agree to meet environmental performance standards and work toward sustainability. Making sure there are strings attached is in the public interest. That's what the Pew Environment Group has suggested. In a letter to US President Barack Obama, Pew Senior Officer Robert Martin noted requests from the pork industry for hundreds of millions of dollars in government assistance to help them through economic downturn and the swine flu crisis. If they're going to get money, he said, "as with the assistance for the auto industry and the financial sectors, this federal assistance should be tied to retooling and improving the swine industry."[84] Producers could receive help if they de-intensified and stopped using antibiotics, or if they adopted manure-management practices like those outlined by waste systems expert Mike Williams of North Carolina. As we heard in Chapter 3 from Dr. Williams, producers are sometimes reluctant to spend money on new methods, no matter how environmentally superior. Governments may need to use financial incentives, or regulatory requirements, or compelling information — carrots, sticks, or sermons.

To encourage sustainable production, authorities need to re-examine resource pricing, as outlined in *Livestock's Long Shadow*. One reason we have more cows, pigs, and chickens than the planet's ecosystems can handle is that the sector has had access to cheap water and land. Natural resources have for years been underpriced — as incentives for agriculture and industry, but also as a legacy of the human tendency to undervalue the natural world. This has given economic advantages to a sector that uses disproportionate amounts of resources.

Water is an example of how more-realistic pricing of resources could increase conservation in livestock production. Water shortages internationally are so serious, and contribute so much to poverty and hunger, that strong policy is needed, says the comprehensive international report *Water for Food, Water for Life*.[85] Each drop of water needs to be made more productive, and the poor need better access. Water needs to be priced higher to encourage conservation in agriculture.[86] Environmental groups and water associations have called for "full-cost pricing,"[87] but ultimately the world will need to rethink entire paradigms for water use in agriculture.[88]

We can make meat using methods that are more ecological, but it will take judicious application of strategies likely to make a difference. Moratoriums are one strategy that has not necessarily done so. The state of North Carolina and the province of Manitoba each currently has a moratorium to limit the growth of the intensive pig industry. That sounds hopeful and suggests that problems from factory hog production are being solved. Yet intensive pig barns remain serious environmental and health issues in both these regions. Furthermore, moratoriums don't necessarily stop industry expansion. In the first decade after the initial 1997 moratorium on hog-industry expansion in North Carolina, half a million more swine were added in the state.[89] That sounds incredible, but according to PigSite, which disseminates information for the global pig industry, exemptions under the legislation allowed not only for some farms to be expanded or reactivated, but even for new farms to be built.[90] An environmental organization similarly reported that the number of factory-farmed pigs in North Carolina continued to increase even during the moratorium.[91] That group, Food and Water Watch, also showed that the number of factory-farmed broiler chickens in the state more than doubled, from 35 million to 80 million, between 1997 and 2007.[92]

As for Lake Winnipeg, it's still dirty. Moratoriums on growth don't necessarily curb pollution from existing farms. And they may not stop construction of farms that got building approvals before the moratoriums took effect. Moratoriums tend not to extend to all CAFOs. In addition, moratoriums can allow operations to expand under some conditions. At a deeper level, such measures have limited effectiveness because they clash with larger policy objectives that encourage big export-oriented business in industrialized countries.

Two Key Strategy Areas: Fewer Antibiotics and More Animal Welfare

What strategies would most help promote sustainable livestock and meat? Of the many possibilities, two stand out that could directly increase sustainability, plus have positive ripple effects. One involves antibiotics (we need less), and the other involves animal welfare (we need more). Policy could put severe limits on antibiotics and enact more stringent requirements for animal welfare.

Antibiotics are a big problem, but an even bigger opportunity for policymakers and society. As outlined earlier, administration of antibiotics is routine in some factory farms and is probably a key factor in the rise of antibiotic resistance. A long and growing list of groups is calling for a re-examination of, and in some cases a ban on, the practice. That list includes the Pew Commission on Industrial Farm Animal Production, the Union of Concerned Scientists, and Keep Antibiotics Working.[93] Antibiotics for livestock have been scaled back significantly in Europe, including in Sweden and Denmark, and the move has been positive for human health. Virtually no Danish swine or chickens have received antibiotics since 2000, in a program that has "been very beneficial in reducing antimicrobial resistance in important food animal reservoirs," according to the World Health Organization.[94]

Meat agribusiness feels the sting of criticism on antibiotics. "The industry is terrified of losing tools on which the whole foundation of their system is based," comments Dr. MacRae. "And they'll fight it tooth and nail." That may be why campaigns to get rid of the practice have made slower progress than the scientific evidence would warrant. Health educators and activists were disappointed[95] when the US Food and Drug Administration backed off its long-time campaign for mandatory cutbacks on major livestock antibiotics.[96] The path to limit livestock antibiotics is certain to be a bumpy one.

Then there is the ethically pressing issue of animal welfare, a moral imperative worthy in itself, but which would also improve sustainability and health. Better animal-welfare systems mean less crowding, which would mean fewer gas emissions and pollution per unit area; lower livestock densities would allow animals to add symbiotically to local ecosystems.

Animal welfare in food production is making headway as some companies make improvements, and some jurisdictions pass animal protection laws either aimed at factory farming or collaterally affecting it. Numerous meat, dairy, and egg companies, plus some governments, are climbing on board. Pork companies are housing pigs in groups rather than in individual cages, which allows them to interact and move about. In Manitoba, at least 85% of pigs are now group-housed, according to the Manitoba Pork Council.[97] Hoop barns, where animals live together under an arched tarp and can nest in straw bedding, are being used for hogs around North America, and they are being tried for cattle too.[98] Some pork producers have pledged to phase out the tiny gestation crates currently used for pregnant sows. A major egg producer, after years of discussions with the Humane Society of the United States, is working toward installing larger cages for hundreds of millions of hens.[99] California, the biggest dairy state in the country, has outlawed the amputation of cows' tails without anesthetic.[100] Michigan passed legislation requiring that farm animals confined in cages have enough room to turn around and fully extend their limbs.[101] However, billions of food animals still live caged and miserable lives, so while new initiatives are laudable, they will need to be monitored and expanded.

Agriculture is at a critical juncture and needs public policy with a vision for short-term incremental shifts as well as long-term and deeper change. If we're going to grow food sustainably and compassionately, we'll need practices and technologies to improve current production methods. But we'll also need the redesign of agricultural systems that promote and encourage such practices as organic farming and low-density production of grassfed livestock. Dr. Ann Clark, retired agriculture professor at the University of Guelph in southern Ontario, agrees that organic farming will be the backbone of sustainable food production, integrating "whatever livestock can be justified on the post-oil landscape."[102] We'll eventually need to address the overarching issues of too many chemicals, too much mechanization, too much corporation concentration, and too little common sense.

Policy Needs to Accommodate Farms Like Sap Bush Hollow

When customers of Sap Bush Hollow Farm want to buy legs or chops from grassfed sheep, the Hayes family isn't allowed to kill and process the animal. Sap Bush does have a small state-licensed slaughterhouse where it is allowed to handle some livestock under some conditions. But for most of their processing, they're required to transport the animals to a US Department of Agriculture facility where the livestock can be inspected and supervised. This means loading the cows and sheep onto trucks and transporting them, which is uncomfortable and frightening for the animals. It also increases — not decreases — the risk of bacterial contamination of the meat. Like other farmers who raise their animals on pasture or grass, Hayes family members are confident that their animals are not harboring harmful amounts of E. coli in their guts. Better to process the animals at home on the farm. But that's not possible without a capital investment to set up a federally approved facility and without adhering to detailed inspection protocols that small farms usually can't afford. Livestock regulations tend to be "one size fits all" and designed for large facilities. That's despite the growing contention that small farms neither need the close inspection nor can they afford it, and that small farms may be healthier for animals and for people.

Sap Bush Hollow has its policy challenges, but day to day, it's a peaceful place to visit, as photographer Seth Joel found when he traveled there to take photographs for this book.[103] His description of the visit made me feel policymakers might want to visit Sap Bush Hollow. Said Mr. Joel:

> "The Hayes family are the most genuine, down-to-earth folks I
> have ever met. It was a pleasure spending the day on the farm.

My only regret was I left my wellies [boots] at home. After the photo session, they invited me in for Sunday lunch. I kicked off my city shoes (now covered with dung) and entered their rustic farm house heated with a wood-burning stove. A small home with views to die for and family memories in every corner. I hung out in the kitchen watching Adele prepare a five-pound leg of lamb, while Shannon was busy at the table making sausages for next week's meal. Shannon's husband Bob was very chatty, and their two young girls filled the house with laughter. Jim was smoking bacon on the front porch and brought in a plate for tasting. Thick chunks flavored with a maple and hickory blend. Very light and not overpowering. I'd say smoked to perfection. I tried not to stuff myself since I knew the lamb was on deck. Dinner was classic. Everything but the cherry tomatoes were home-raised on the farm. Leg of lamb. Green beans. Potatoes and acorn squash. The roast was tender and juicy with a rich honest taste. Good thing I'm a meat eater."

Solutions May Require International Cooperation

An international treaty on meat and dairy reduction is one suggestion that's been put on the table, served up by the formidable European animal-welfare organization Compassion in World Farming (CIWF).[104] A high-level treaty might sound fanciful, but this organization and its officials are not simply dreamers. CIWF and its employees have been working for decades to augment animal welfare in Europe and around the world. Among their achievements is a prestigious awards program for food producers that meet high animal-welfare standards, which is improving the lives of hundreds of millions of farm animals.[105] CIWF also produces valuable educational and informational materials. I visited the organization several years ago at its office, which is a short train ride south of London. I somehow expected a few advocates in a basement office, but found an entire floor of an office building full of people working effectively for animal welfare.

CIWF officials believe that a multi-country agreement is one possible strategy for dealing with the environmental, welfare, and health problems of livestock and meat, as Joyce D'Silva told me.[106] Ms. D'Silva is former chief executive of the organization and is now director of public affairs there. Such a treaty could be negotiated among governments, she said, and could set fair meat reduction targets for high-consumption countries while allowing low-consumption countries to increase their intake. As part of that, all countries would work to enhance local small-scale livestock farming.

It's hard to know how the world might tackle the meat problem without such multilateral projects. The discussion needs traction globally, which it is starting to get. The United Nations Food and Agriculture Organization has proclaimed the need for action.[107] The Intergovernmental Panel on Climate Change is well aware of the contribution of livestock to greenhouse gases.[108] And the UN Environmental Program (UNEP) has said current levels of meat production and consumption may be ecologically impossible long term. Citizens have responded on the UNEP website with comments including: "Simply eating less meat will mean using less energy, creating less deforestation, living more healthily and loving all sentient beings. ...I think a good tip would be having people eat less meat and try to go vegetarian. ...The easiest thing anyone can do is eat less meat."[109]

Finding solutions may require global collaboration, which is the basis of the "contraction and convergence" proposal discussed earlier that has been advanced by international scientists.[110] Such a program would be part of a broader "portfolio strategy" to mitigate climate change, minimize pollution, and otherwise improve environmental health, as Australian scientist Dr. Anthony McMichael and others have written.[111]

Smart people will need to talk. Courageous people will need to recognize that livestock have roamed roughshod, not only over Earth, but over policy. Visionary cooperation is needed for solutions to one of the pressing problems of our time.

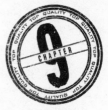

SOCIETY CAN OVERCOME THE BARRIERS

Social Norms Can Shift

When did it happen that animal products became part of every dish? On a research trip, I was at the airport of a major city and looking to find a light snack for the plane. Approaching the healthiest-looking deli counter, I scanned the options. The sandwiches were uniformly filled with conventional beef, turkey, or tuna. Even the salads, all four on the menu, contained a heaping portion of chicken, and one had bacon as well. The desserts didn't seem to contain meat, but each one was mostly cream or cheese.

Today, even sandwiches and salads have been swept up in the meat binge. Our menus are in stark contrast to traditional suppers that consisted of a core food such as rice, a fringe item such as a sauce, plus a legume, according to food anthropologist Sidney Mintz. Now, entire meals are often described only by the animal products, as in "we're having chicken for dinner," and by researchers as "M + S + 2V" which stands for "meat plus a staple plus two vegetables." When that equation applies to billions of people, it can add up to major problems for the environment and public health.[1]

Regular intake of meat is so pervasive a part of our culture that we take it for granted. Large-scale meat consumption is reinforced through grocery stores and restaurants, in cooking schools and food magazines, and in gourmet and "foodie" circles. And the reinforcement is not just because our meat-based diets are so interesting and varied. Many of us settle on a handful of favorite meals and eat them over and over. Today, many of those meals are based on animal products. It's become a social norm, one of those unwritten expectations that guide our behavior.

Yet we can establish new food norms that minimize the meat. Yes, we are genetically predisposed to enjoy fatty and high-calorie meals, but the evidence shows that most of us would enjoy better health with less. Yes, we like the sensory experiences we associate with meat, but some of those tastes come from sauces and spices that could just as well accessorize plant-based meals. Yes, we feel that meat is a label of status, but we probably have higher priorities. Yes, we've been told that beef, pork, and chicken are necessary, but low-meat and plant-based diets provide plenty of nutrients and all we need for health.[2]

Even long-held ideas on this are amenable to solutions. Flesh foods have historically represented virility and power and been perceived as important to human growth and progress.[3] Meat companies are hoping that's still the case, as I saw in a recent television ad in which a young man is seated in front of a plate-sized steak. He finishes it off to hearty congratulations from his friends, and an authoritative voice-over reminds us that beef "makes men act like men."[4] But recent surveys in Europe suggest such positive associations with meat may be in decline. Researchers Erik de Bakker and Hans Dagevos of the Netherlands Agricultural Economics Research Institute conducted a consumer investigation indicating "there might be a shift going on in the cultural image and appreciation of meat: that meat is less a token of masculinity" and less uniformly desirable than it used to be.[5]

As discussed in Chapter 6, social norms can change precisely because they're social. The beliefs and perceptions that drive the meat binge are not entirely inborn; they are amplified — and in some cases created — through agribusiness marketing, advertising, and lobbying, as I'll show later in this chapter. But alternative messages can be spread, and initiatives can offer a different point of view. Project CHEF (Cook Healthy Edible Food) is one program in my hometown that does just that. Barb Finley and her staff give hands-on lessons at elementary schools, teaching children to prepare dishes such as granola, Greek salad, apple raita, and pizza with whole-grain crust and lots of vegetables.[6] These educators use small amounts of cheese and a little chicken stock, but aim to introduce young people to healthy and environmentally friendly meals. "We are such a meat-eating society," says Ms. Finley. "At Project CHEF we try to open children's eyes to the many other choices that are open to people."[7] It's a small example, but it's one being played out across the United States, Canada, and elsewhere as citizens look to eat in ways that are good for health and ecosystems.

Social norms can change, especially when a novel idea is evidence-based and powerful and people are exposed to it for a time. Even so, cultural shifts don't happen overnight or smoothly. According to one analysis of social movements,[8] there is first a period in which critics

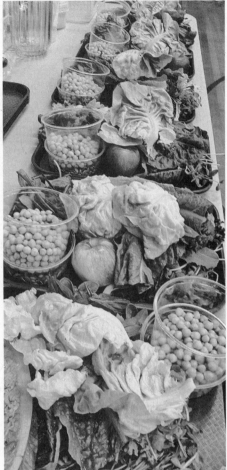

Credit: Project CHEF

Salad ingredients ready for schoolchildren to use, in the program run by Project CHEF (Cook Healthy Edible Food) discussed in Chapter 6.

publicly demonstrate the weakness of existing systems and face strong opposition from the populace and special interests. As the new idea spreads and slowly gains acceptance, conditions ripen for change and a single event can trigger a leap forward. That's what happened when Rosa Parks was arrested in Alabama in 1955 for refusing to move to the back of the bus, an action now viewed as catalytic to the subsequent progress in legislation on civil rights. It's what happened to the World

Trade Organization when demonstrators so disrupted its 1999 Seattle meetings as to amplify public skepticism about its controversial agenda of worldwide liberalization of trade.[9] As author Malcolm Gladwell has written, change can sweep across a population once a "tipping point" is reached.[10] Ideas can act like viruses that spread and reach a critical mass, exploding into epidemics that infect whole communities. Even then, social change is often erratic and chaotic rather than a linear movement toward another way. Two steps forward, one step back, as they say. The "eat less meat" movement is at an early stage, still contending with deeply held beliefs and social structures that support industrial production and heavy consumption. But the norms are ripe for change.

Meat-Eaters, Vegans, and Everyone Else Can Be on the Same Team

Optimism is useful for anyone who's contemplating the meat problem, which was a good reason to attend the first National Conference to End Factory Farming, held in October 2011, near Washington, DC. The event was a statement of hope that it's just a matter of time before we develop food systems that are more sustainable and compassionate.[11] Hundreds of us were moved to tears as speakers described small livestock farmers living in poverty in the shadow of animal factories, water and air pollution moving directly from CAFOs to families' homes, and stories like one about Rosie the pig who was rescued and nurtured at Farm Sanctuary where she was finally able to indulge her maternal instinct and live a natural life.[12] Yet the tone of the sessions was confident about our ability to transform intensive livestock production.

As was evident at the conference, there is a swelling group of motivated people and organizations seeking to transform livestock production that is neither sustainable nor compassionate. Of the attendees, some were vegans, some were meat-eaters, and many fell in the spectrum in between. Of the organizations, some focused on conserving ecosystems, others on improving conditions for animals, and others on the health of individuals and communities. All were brought together by Farm Sanctuary, an impressive organization that is at the center of these issues. Farm Sanctuary rescues abused farm animals and nurtures

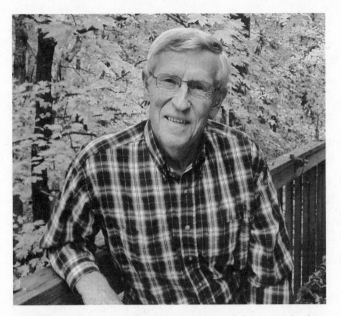

John Ikerd, professor emeritus of agricultural economics in Missouri, suggests that everyone from vegans to meat-eaters can work together against intensive livestock systems, and for food production that is compassionate and sustainable.

them to health at its three locations in upstate New York and California. They also educate the public and advocate widely for better animal protection.

One stirring speaker at the conference was John Ikerd, professor emeritus of agricultural economics at the University of Missouri. He has spent more than 30 years teaching people how to engage thoughtfully in animal agriculture, and he believes it is morally defensible to raise animals for food. But he is passionately opposed to the takeover of meat production by factory farming. "CAFOs are the epitome of everything that is wrong with the industrial food system," he told a conference session. Promoted to government and the general public as an efficient way to produce meat, CAFOs don't even produce more meat than smaller farms did, he said. CAFOs are purportedly a rural development strategy. "But the rural communities end up being worse off than they were. Studies invariably show that communities without CAFOs are better places to live."[13]

Dr. Ikerd was raised on a small Missouri dairy farm where hunting and fishing were part of life and survival. He was aware that animals had feelings and intrinsic worth and value as part of the natural world. But animals were also sources of sustenance for him and his family. "I've been thinking about these issues all my life," he told me in an interview. "Every living thing lives by consuming the remains of other once-living things. And humans aren't the only ones that don't always wait for them to die first."

Over the years, Dr. Ikerd has watched as representatives of animal factories approached rural communities proposing intensive livestock facilities. They would invariably paint opponents as outsiders and radical environmentalists. "They tear rural communities apart with dissent between proponents and opponents. They tell people there are no alternatives to factory farming, but there are."[14]

We can develop sustainable alternatives, according to Dr. Ikerd, if CAFO opponents work together — everyone, across the omnivorous spectrum. "We're not going to resolve our basic philosophical differences, but we all want to end factory farming. We all agree that animals should be treated with respect and dignity, and that CAFOs are bad for people, for animals, and for rural communities."[15] It was a widespread sentiment at the conference. As Dr. Ikerd put it: "We've got to focus on our common aims."

Political Impediments Can Be Addressed

Solving the meat problem is going to take persistence, because most officials would rather steer clear. That was made evident by the UN FAO when it decried the lack of public policy on the issue.[16] I've also learned first-hand that authorities, whether national, state, or city, are reluctant parties to the discussion. On one occasion, I'd been given approval to speak to a food security committee in a large municipality, where I laid out reasons for the city to consider supporting Meatless Monday. But the most spirited response, from an intensive livestock farmer on the committee, was to grill and roast me for trying to drive meat producers out of business. At another time and place, I had attended a forum for politicians to discuss residents' environmental ideas. But even when

data-collectors revealed that the most numerous food-related suggestion was that the city encourage lower meat consumption, politicians
kept the discussion on safer ground. Perhaps they were shy because
many of the suggestions promoted veganism, a diet with no animal
products at all. No matter how it is framed, though, for most authorities, the meat problem is at the bottom of the to-do list.

Contentious and complex, the topic is perceived by elected officials
as a no-win issue that is bound to alienate both producers and consumers, most of them regular meat-eaters and all of them voters. So-called
high-value foods are a symbol of the good life, especially when they're
priced within most people's reach. "Meat goes to the heart of policymakers' notions of progress," write researchers Tim Lang, Michelle Wu,
and Martin Caraher.[17] And few leaders wish to challenge voters' aspi-
rations. Informing people they'll need to cut back on steak or bacon
may feel like telling children there's no Santa. "Meat is seen by policymakers as an issue to leave in the 'too hard to deal with' box," observe
the researchers, "and to 'leave for my successor to deal with.'"[18] Official
distaste for the topic is compounded by its reputation as a polarized
tug-of-war between meat-eaters and vegetarians. Add to that the con-
voluted nature of the problem, and you've got a low priority.

Even citizen groups promoting sustainable food often sideline the
meat problem. Sometimes it's because they're not sure where to start.
But often, it's to avoid aligning themselves with vegetarian activists
or alienating agribusiness. One food-security organizer in a major
metropolis told me he avoids raising the meat topic because it might
antagonize producers.

The political challenges start with the economic ocean in which
we all swim. As discussed in Chapter 6, the international rules of the
World Trade Organization (WTO) facilitate industrial production and
encourage large-scale, cross-border flows of goods. Global trade agreements assume continued expansion and growth. So doing less of anything, or doing it locally, doesn't really fit. I asked an acquaintance the
other day how his work was going with his government job promoting local and sustainable food. There's very little budget, he confided.
Elected officials like to reassure citizens and farmers that they're on

the side of local food, and theoretically they may be. But they're often limited in their ability to promote it because of commitments to industry and export. Global trade is controversial, especially the inclusion of agriculture under the WTO, and some argue that food should be excluded or at least treated differently from other goods.[19] Olivier de Schutter, UN Special Rapporteur on the Right to Food, has openly challenged the WTO and recommended a different approach to trade policy that will be needed if the world is going to feed itself.[20] Meanwhile, governments support industrial livestock and meat as integral to their promotion of trade.

Another political barrier to addressing the meat problem is that livestock governance tends to be a jumble of rules and regulations at numerous government levels and departments with, as the saying goes, too many cooks spoiling the broth. When it comes to regulating factory farming, ironically, there can be so many officials, departments, and agencies that paralysis can ensue. Over-involvement can hog-tie the parties into under-involvement. In Manitoba, for example, the intensive livestock industry is governed at three levels and by two or more federal departments and numerous provincial ones. There are at least 18 pieces of provincial legislation bearing on hog production, from *The Environment Act* to *The Planning Act*.[21] The industry is governed by laws or regulations overseen by Manitoba Conservation, Manitoba Agriculture, Food and Rural Initiatives, and Water Stewardship, Health, and Intergovernmental Affairs.

In many jurisdictions, when a decision, regulation, or enforcement is bound to make people and organizations unhappy (especially powerful ones), lines of authority can become muddy. Because it's not always clear who's supposed to make a decision about waste management facilities or meat inspection or where factory farms can locate, there is sometimes competition — not only for the right to make decisions, but for the right not to make them. On antibiotics, for example, officials have been known to shift responsibility to avoid having to deal with this touchy topic.[22] Government officials are sometimes in a quandary, observed one researcher, "internally divided on the issue of ILOs (intensive livestock operations) and lacking sufficient information or jurisdictional authority to practice effective environmental democracy."[23]

Intensifying the trouble are competing priorities within governments and even departments. One division can be charged with cleaning up health and the environment, and another with promoting and encouraging industry. The US Department of Agriculture, which has responsibility for promoting sales of food commodities, "is hardly likely to issue advice — to eat less meat, for example — that conflicts with its assigned mission," says nutrition expert Dr. Nestle in her book *What to Eat*.[24] Manitoba's Clean Environment Commission, when grappling with hog-barn pollution, observed that "an inevitable conflict arises within government when it has the roles of both promoting and regulating an industry."[25] Competing interests are a fact of life, but an unfortunate one when government systems are set up to pit economic growth against environment and health.

Competing interests and uncertain responsibility for food safety were partly blamed for the mad cow crisis in the UK during the 1990s.[26] Food is so important, and its administration so Byzantine, that it's not easy to determine how responsibility should be allocated to allow for real action on big problems.[27]

Compounding the political challenges is regulation of intensive livestock that has been evolving toward ever-higher levels. It used to be that a rural municipality would have a lot to say about whether a factory farm came to town. But changes to planning laws have eroded local decision-making and disempowered municipalities. Other kinds of legislation have made recourse difficult for individuals who are adversely affected by intensive production. Canadian environmentalist Elizabeth Brubaker, executive director of Environment Probe, has documented the trend away from local control. In her book *Greener Pastures*, Ms. Brubaker suggested that pollution is increasingly the purview of provincial authorities that use "right to farm" legislation to justify agricultural pollution because it is "normal."[28] An evolution of decision-making to higher levels also makes it difficult for environmentalists to effectively question industry practices, which helps protect jurisdictions' reputations as safe for investment. When your local town council is making a decision about food systems, you can attend a meeting and speak up. But when a decision is being made at state, provincial, or federal levels, it's difficult to get your voice heard.

All these realities make it difficult to alter the status quo on industrial livestock production. Business as usual is supported by international trade agreements, pro-industry attitudes in governments, unclear decision-making authority, pressure from producers, and uncertainty from consumers. These are among the reasons that US President Barack Obama, who understands the issues and has vowed to tackle the problems of factory farming,[29] has a challenge on his hands. It's no wonder politicians, at any level of governance, steer clear. But what's life without a challenge? The meat issue is polarized, contentious, and complex, so let's get to work.

Corporate Influence Can Be Questioned

Excessive power of the few over the many is a theme for our time. It's the underpinning for democratic movements all over the world. It's what sparked the dramatic Occupy protests in the autumn of 2011. Quantified by growing income inequality, the problem is so severe that even the mainstream Organization for Economic Cooperation and Development has issued a report arguing that inequalities are socially corrosive and bad for everyone.[30] Meanwhile, the structure of the meat sector is one example of concentrated power.

Decades of industrially oriented farm policy and corporate mergers have allowed a handful of companies to control much of our food, as discussed in Chapter 5. Wenonah Hauter, executive director of the Washington-based environmental group Food and Water Watch, believes limits are needed on corporate concentration in food and agriculture.[31] Organizations like hers are heartened that Washington is concerned, as demonstrated by the fact that the US Department of Justice held a series of public workshops in 2010 to hear people's views on competition and anti-trust enforcement issues in agriculture.[32]

Corporations and their trade groups work hard to shape policy. One way they do this is through lobbying. "Livestock lobbies have been able to exert an over-proportional influence on public policies, to protect their interests," says the FAO.[33] Industry representatives work the halls of power to present the agribusiness point of view on issues from animal welfare to drug policy to environmental regulation to taxation. Trade groups represent producers of beef, pork, chicken, turkeys, eggs, and dairy, and also the meat sector as a whole. The Animal Agriculture Alliance spends millions "to communicate the importance of modern animal agriculture to consumers and the media," says its website.[34] Aware that not everyone agrees, at a recent stakeholders summit, the industry provided tips to companies on how to identify "potential employee imposters/activists."[35] Groups such as the Canadian Meat Council have energetic agendas that include lobbying to ensure that legislation and practices help, rather than hinder, meat-packing and processing businesses. It promotes producers' viewpoints on food safety, nutrition, and animal issues, and it says it is pushing for further approval in Canada of antimicrobials for livestock.[36]

Lobbying is aggressive in the United States, where a coalition of industry groups deploys large numbers of lawyers and representatives to protect their interests.[37] Their influence been documented by Dr. Nestle, who has shown that US dietary guidelines have been affected by industry. For example, when the guidelines were being revised in the 1970s based on nutritional and health data, the government was set to recommend that consumers reduce their intake of meat and other foods high in fat, sugar, and salt.[38] This generated a storm of protest. Soon, the draft recommendations were diluted to the point of essentially advising consumers to eat more animal products. As Dr. Nestle records, the phrase "reduce consumption of meat" was replaced with "choose meats, poultry, and fish which will reduce saturated fat intake."[39] Later government recommendations defaulted to an even more upbeat "choose lean meat."[40] When suggestions get sufficiently vague, they have less bite.

Questioning corporate influence also requires recognition of business involvement in academic research. Scientific research today is often industry-funded, and meat corporations (like pharmaceutical companies) have economic and cultural power partly through such involvement. That may sound surprising, because university research is supposed to be objective. But many universities and faculty researchers accept and even solicit corporate money, including from the meat industry. And while funding sources shouldn't affect results, it appears that when corporations pay, academic reports are more prone to have a flattering tinge. Investigators at Yale University conducted an overview of biomedical studies to demonstrate that industry-sponsored research is "significantly more likely to reach conclusions that were favorable to the sponsor" than is independent research.[41] Why wouldn't it be similar on food issues? Dr. Nestle cites the telling example of research into soft drinks and childhood obesity: "Independent studies almost invariably find an association between habitual consumption of soft drinks and obesity," she says. "By contrast, industry-sponsored studies almost never do."[42]

Industry involvement in academic research was noted by the Pew Commission in its report on industrial animal production. When commission researchers approached agribusiness for information, it encountered "responses ranging from open hostility to wary cooperation."[43] The commission reported instances of academics being warned that if they assisted the Pew group, their research money could dry up. "We found significant influence by the industry at every turn," wrote Pew Executive Director Robert Martin, "in academic research, agriculture policy development, government regulation, and enforcement."[44] All these efforts converged on the aim of encouraging consumers not to eat less, but more.

The phenomenon of corporate funding of research is familiar to activists such as Rick Dove in North Carolina. "When I first started this work," he said, "I thought university researchers were pure and clean."[45] Now he says that if you're looking for the whole story, you need to find research that doesn't just tell the corporate one.

Questioning corporate influence also means questioning advertising and promotion. As a metaphorical first step, we could question the color of pork. It's officially classified as a red meat by agriculture and food officials,[46] but a successful advertising campaign by the National Pork Board called it "the other white meat."[47] Meat and dairy companies are fighting to keep consumers thinking positively, and favorable perceptions of white meat have figuratively turned pork a lighter shade of pink.

Industrial meat producers and their trade groups rely on marketing and public relations, so multi-million dollar advertising campaigns announce: "Beef: It's What's for Dinner,"[48] and in Australia a few years ago: "Red Meat: We Were Meant to Eat It."[49] Food companies spend many millions each year to coax people to eat more of their products, and meat companies are part of it. One large company spent tens of millions to urge you to buy meats with their company's logo.[50] Because advertising works, industries ensure constant funding for their marketing campaigns. In US beef and pork industries, a compulsory "checkoff" program requires producers to pay into marketing funds — for example, beef producers pay $1 per head of cattle — to promote flesh foods.[51] Industry websites funded by the Beef Checkoff[52] and the Pork Checkoff[53] list the many activities being paid for by producers' checkoff money. Though dissident producers have complained about the cost and compulsory nature of the program, industry groups have prevailed and gather tens of millions of dollars annually to market meat.[54]

For shaping norms, there's nothing like education, so agribusiness also provides instructional units for schoolteachers. Often too busy to develop their own teaching materials, teachers sometimes rely on ready-made ones from industry. So Manitoba children can read colorful fact sheets from the pork council to help them develop positive feelings about pork.[55] The Dairy Council of California distributes educational materials for children — some as young as kindergarten age — that provide fun activities like Color My Pizza.[56]

Lobbying for government influence, funding research, and advertising to shape consumer beliefs are all part of the reach of food corporations that already have power simply by virtue of their size. It's up to us to question the messages and the system and the food choices these encourage, and ask whether these are wise.

We Can Educate Ourselves About the Meat Problem

When we imagine how we might produce fewer greenhouse gases, we think of limiting our driving or flying. When we imagine ways our community could decrease water pollution, we think of enforcing regulations on heavy industry. When we imagine how we might dine more healthfully, we think of consuming less soda and fewer potato chips.

When we imagine countering animal abuse, we think of getting tough on practices such as dog-fighting. But while such responses are helpful, we can often do more for the environment, for health, and for animals by addressing the issue of excessive industrial meat production and consumption.

Animal welfare is a poignant example of the need to educate ourselves about meat production. We're compassionate people, and we are pained when we hear about pets that have been abused or dogs that are forced to battle for human entertainment. Yet in "raw units of suffering," no animal-welfare issue compares to intensive production of animals for food, said Wayne Pacelle to the National Conference to End Factory Farming. President and chief executive of the Humane Society of the United States, Mr. Pacelle noted that dog-fighting engenders public outcries and is illegal in numerous states, though the number of dogs affected is small. Meanwhile, 8–9 billion animals are killed each year in the United States for food — most of them after short and unhappy lives in intensive farms.[57]

Environmental and health problems, similarly, get blamed on cars or fried foods, even when massive meat production and consumption is clearly a substantial contributor. But we can educate ourselves to recognize the role of meat.

Even government authorities need to be informed, since they are often unaware of the consequences of modern meat. Some official neglect of the issue is conscious and deliberate, such as when better food production systems are politically difficult or costly. But according to the FAO, "there is a lack of understanding about the nature and extent of livestock's impact on the environment, among producers, consumers, and policymakers alike."[58]

Among consumers, many have heard or read that meat production is hard on the environment, but they don't have enough information to be sure. Even knowledgeable citizens can easily be confused by disparate and seemingly contradictory messages about what's good to eat for health or the environment. Then there is uncertainty about whether consumers need to become vegetarian (they don't) to address the problems.

Chefs, especially those who teach, are well placed to educate people about solutions. Chef Laura Lee of the Napa Valley Cooking School confirmed for me in an interview that she frequently contends with misconceptions from students and diners that meat is necessary at every meal. She is helping change that, by teaching the importance of sustainability in food. In an e-mail to me, she wrote:

"As you are aware, Americans are trained from an early age that animal products are a very important part of a daily diet. Add to that the media push for fast-food chains that make people believe that hamburger, fries and a shake should make up one of your three meals a day. It is not hard to understand why Americans are obese and addicted to nutritionally void food and prescriptions instead of healthy lifestyle as a means to feeling good. Here at the Napa Valley Cooking School we do not believe or teach that animal products are the core of every meal. Eating meat is not a problem, it is the quantity and quality of everything that we put in our mouths that we are focused on. In addition, we train our students in proper preparation of a variety of vegetarian diets including vegan, raw, lacto-ovo and pescatarian."[59]

As we become informed, we will better understand how to shift toward sustainability and help others do the same. Food policy expert Rod MacRae has studied reasons that farmers resist using chemical-free practices such as organic agriculture. One set of reasons is financial. Farmers are understandably anxious about money in a new and unfamiliar system of growing and marketing food. But another barrier is farmers' concern they won't have access to information and support. They lack mentors and people with expertise on whom they can call, says Dr. MacRae.[60] For farmers, chefs, food producers, government officials, and the rest of us, increased knowledge and accurate information will facilitate change.

Citizens Can Prevail

Rural residents have been meeting around kitchen tables for decades, organizing against intensive livestock production. And sometimes they prevail, as happened a decade ago in the case of the hog barn that never got built.

Farmer and activist Fred Tait[61] tells the story that unfolded in Portage La Prairie, a small city in southern Manitoba. A pork corporation had applied to build an intensive operation there. The provincial government's technical review team gave its approval, despite protests from local citizens, who had analyzed the proposal and found indications that the barn could become a serious polluter. The proposed manure lagoons appeared inadequate to hold the projected amounts of waste. As well, the company document claimed there would be a cold storage facility to hold "mortalities" (dead pigs), but the blueprints showed no such facility.[62]

Mr. Tait, who was part of the citizen group, has never seen a provincial review team reject a hog-barn proposal, no matter how many community and environmental problems critics might predict.[63] Review teams might point out concerns, but rarely, if ever, does one reject a proposal. The citizens mustered their energy for the next stage of the process and appeared at municipal hearings to present their analysis. Local officials rejected the proposal, and the hog barn was escorted out of town before it ever settled in.

Citizens can have some influence, and local governments can retain some control. But in most cases, ordinary people don't have the time or resources needed to analyze corporate proposals. Meanwhile, higher levels of government aren't necessarily motivated to prioritize environmental enforcement. They tend to favor intensive livestock facilities, whose voluminous production suits government economic objectives, and whose owners sit in offices far from the smell. Mr. Tait relates how, when citizens asked provincial reviewers why the flawed proposal was endorsed, they received a letter saying that review team members "are not required to check the proponent's material for accuracy."[64] In other words, regulators could accept the contentions of the corporate applicant as fact. Other farmers and environmentalists have expressed similar complaints. The National Farmers' Union has submitted a brief to the Province saying technical review committees are not sufficiently independent of either industry or government.[65]

In the meantime, citizens are questioning the wisdom of intensive factory farming and working to popularize the notion that there is a better way. "Organized local opposition to factory hog-barn developments is one of the most significant recent signs of political life in rural Canada," according to Dr. Roger Epp, an Alberta political scientist.[66] These citizens aren't just against something, he points out. They have a positive vision:

"That vision is about a different countryside than the one that governments and corporate investors apparently have in mind. It is about a different rural economy — less extractive, more resilient, and more respectful of people's livelihoods, local knowledge, and environmental limits. It's about a different food system — more decentralized, and therefore safer and more sustainable, than the continental and global one that is being shaped by a small cluster of vertically integrated processing giants. And not least, it is about a different democratic politics in which real authority is restored to communities. The stakes are that high, and they unite rural people in Canada with those in North Carolina and Iowa, Mexico and Poland."[67]

That dream gives me hope that livestock and meat can be pried out of the "too hard to deal with" box. Challenging it may be, but the meat problem has potential solutions. Governments have policy options (some of which were laid out in Chapter 8) for supporting sustainable producers and encouraging better consumption. Civil society organizations and individual citizens can make the meat problem a priority, calling for changes to factory farming and a widespread consumer reappraisal of the place of flesh foods in our diets and our lives.

As we improve our understanding of the meat problem, we can also work with producers. I said earlier that people who advocate for lower meat consumption are accused of trying to put livestock farmers out of business. While we don't want anyone to lose a job or a livelihood, it's true that a trend to lower meat consumption would affect production systems. There could be disappointment among those who took a risk with their money and their lives, in good faith, to go into business providing food that consumers wanted. This happens in other indus-tries, too, from forestry to mining to personal computing, as consumer tastes and economies shift. There's no easy solution to the frightening and dislocating aspects of social change

But a trend toward more sustainable agriculture could ultimately result in more jobs, not fewer. Growing plants and livestock organically and ecologically is more labor-intensive than growing food under an industrial model. As people develop more moderate attitudes toward meat consumption, society will need to help producers transition to more sustainable practices and new jobs in a new kind of agriculture.

"The world's livestock sector is at the junction of several of the great environmental and moral issues of the modern age. This includes the urgent issues of food security, under-nutrition and its health consequences, environmental degradation, exacerbation of global climate change and concern for animal welfare.... With current production methods, the projected level of meat consumption over coming decades is not environmentally sustainable."

— A. McMichael and A. Butler, "Environmentally Sustainable and Equitable Meat Consumption in a Climate Change World," in *The Meat Crisis*, edited by J. D'Silva and J. Webster, Earthscan, 2010, p. 187.

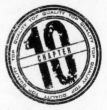

CONSUMERS WILL HELP
LOWER THE STAKES

The Meat Problem Is Amenable to Solutions

We can eat in ways that are good for the planet and ourselves, and that don't consign animals to lives of misery. And we can do it without giving up on animal products. But the change will require decisions to be made by each of us as individuals, by our communities, and by our governments. It will also require the kinds of personal and policy strategies outlined in this book, and summarized here:

Personal Strategies for Consumers:
- Make the decision to decrease your intake of animal products.
- Find sustainable sources.
- Minimize wastage of food, especially meat, fish, and dairy products.
- Support organizations working for fewer and better animal products.
- Don't worry who eats meat and who doesn't; work with everyone.
- Ask restaurants and grocers for more meatless meal items and for more organic and eco-labeled animal products.
- Tell elected officials you want food policy that supports sustainably and compassionately produced animal-source foods.

Policy Strategies for Governments:

- Develop visionary food policy, prioritizing environment and public health.
- Strengthen laws to decrease livestock pollution and gas emissions.
- Place stricter limits on antibiotics and other chemicals in livestock.
- Implement tighter standards for farm animal welfare.
- Require livestock producers to pay full costs for inputs and cleanup.
- Limit corporate concentration in agribusiness.
- Initiate public education for citizens, food producers, and policymakers on healthy production and consumption of animal products.

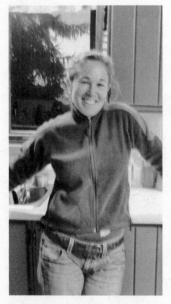

Colleen Ross in the kitchen on her farm in southern Ontario, Canada. By taking practical responsibility for food and also being politically active, Ms. Ross practices food sovereignty.

We Can Get Inspired

Tramping around a muddy farmyard with Colleen Ross and her chickens and sheep was energizing for me. She's the southern Ontario organic farmer introduced in Chapter 5, with whom I had the pleasure to visit. Reflecting on her ideas, I came to feel that we can all contribute to better food systems in ways that could be summarized as: "get into the kitchen, get out to the farm, and get involved."

Colleen gets into the kitchen. She's an excellent cook, as evidenced by a bowl of her minestrone soup. During harvest, she gathers peppers, tomatoes, and other vegetables, along with rye and soy, then preserves food for future months. "I dehydrate, I ferment, I freeze, I can. I'm into food preservation for my own personal food security. You've got to practice food sovereignty."[1]

If you've read this far, you're probably contemplating practicing more of your own food sovereignty. I'd like to say it won't take much time or effort. There are convenient ways to access healthy foods. You don't need to spend all day, and you don't need to make everything from scratch. You do not need to turn your life upside down. But buying fresh vegetables and preparing them does take more energy than ordering a pizza or heating a can of stew. It takes effort to rethink habits, and to eat well. For Colleen, healthy food is worth the trouble.

Just as Colleen gets into the kitchen, so Jim and Adele Hayes, and their daughter Shannon and her family, get out to the farm. They get out there every day because it's where they live, but we can too, either physically or by proxy, through local food markets. But just as it takes effort to shift toward making and consuming healthy food, getting out to farms isn't necessarily easy or uncomplicated. To drive to Sap Bush Hollow Farm, about 50 minutes west of Albany, New York, you need to follow the website directions that warn: "Now pay attention, because you don't want to get lost out here!"[2] It's a metaphor for the reality that eating better takes commitment. Especially for city people who are accustomed to buying meals canned or wrapped in cellophane, we need to go to some trouble, make some adjustments, find some time. Getting out to the farm also requires a financial decision, because you may pay more than you would for factory-produced chicken and pork. But, as part of the project, you'll be eating less meat.

Farmers like the Hayes family have told me they want and need to meet their customers. One of the problems for sustainable farmers is that, however skilled and productive they may be, they're often not expert at marketing themselves and their food. As long as advertising and distribution systems are geared toward industrial operations, it helps if you and I get out of town once in a while to buy direct. I met more than one small-scale farmer who integrates livestock into crop production and ends up with more meat than could easily be sold. It's pristine stuff — chemical-free and grass- and pasture-raised. But farmers don't always have the marketing channels to potential customers.

Because it's not always easy to literally get out to the farm, you can also do so figuratively by identifying discerning neighborhood grocers. There are farmers' markets and local food networks to explore. Many cities have healthy-food delivery services such as one in Texas called

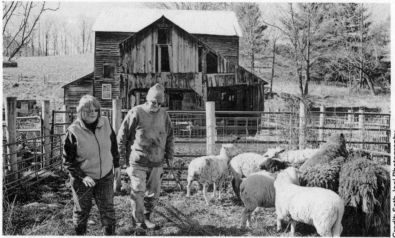

Adele and Jim Hayes on their farm, where they produce chemical-free meat from animals raised in a natural and healthy environment.

Greenling.[3] Customers sign up and receive regular bins that can include meat, dairy, and eggs, in reusable cold packs that keep the food chilly for hours, even in the hot southern sun. Customers receive fresh produce and other grocery items, grown and raised organically or with methods judged by the company to be local and sustainable.[4] Your city or community almost certainly has a system for organic produce delivery, or some program to get you out to the local countryside or to bring its food to you.

As committed people get into the kitchen and out to the farm, Conner Ingram is getting involved in his own way. A 13-year-old elementary school student in West Vancouver, Conner has been thinking about food since he saw the documentary *Super Size Me*[5] when he was seven years old. Yes, 7. Seeing the movie made him question the wisdom of fast food and commonplace eating habits. Conner's interest was further sparked when he saw the movie *Food Inc.*,[6] examining the environmental and health sides of factory farming. So when one of his teachers asked students to do a class presentation on any topic, Conner chose to look at meat, the way it is produced, and the amounts we eat. He was concerned about antibiotics, chemicals, and pollution, about animal welfare, the environment, and health, and he wanted to educate others.

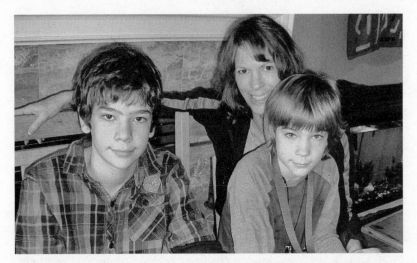

Conner Ingram decided to eat only sustainably and compassionately produced animal products, and educates other young people to do the same. L to R: Conner Ingram, mother Linda Watt, and Conner's brother Miles Ingram.

Conner recalls that, on presentation day, he gave his speech and showed computer slides to fellow students, and "everybody was completely shocked," he said. "Especially me, because I electrocuted myself." His cable was frayed, sparks went flying, and Conner got a jolt, another metaphor for the experience. Conner has not become vegetarian, but tries to choose animal products that are humanely and healthfully produced. His mother and the rest of the family are on board, and generally avoid conventional meat. "It has changed what I eat. ... I'll eat a homemade burger," says Conner, "but not the fast-food kind." Family members agree that this kind of conscious eating can make life a little more difficult. Good meat costs more. They're no longer willing to eat hotdogs. And when they're up the mountain skiing for the day, or out of town, it can be hard to find good food. But Conner is involved, and he feels it's got to be done.[7]

How did a 13-year-old get interested in such topics? What was he doing at the age of seven viewing a topical documentary? What is it in individuals that drive them to care and to act? In Conner's case, his parents are filmmakers who often watch documentaries and include

Conner and his younger brother Miles. Conner is bright, inquisitive, and thoughtful. All these factors have laid the groundwork for his concern and involvement.

For the rest of us, and for society, what makes for change? How can any of us, and all of us, make the commitment to better food? We need to lay our own groundwork, then follow up at personal levels and at policy ones. We need to be informed and inspired, as we can be by people like Colleen, Jim, Adele, Shannon, and Conner. They're taking action, and so can we.

High Steaks Is a Theme for Our Time

The steaks are high, with global meat consumption at all-time high levels and livestock production creating problems for the environment, health, and communities. The meat problem raises questions about how we eat, how we treat people and animals, and how we choose to live. It raises questions about our values. As suggested in the Introduction, meat is a mighty theme for us as individuals and societies.

Addressing the problem is essential to food sustainability and to satisfying the hunger among us for responsible consumption. The meat issue can work hand in hand with other aspects of the food movement, including the crucial transition to more locally produced food, and the move toward organic and chemical-free agriculture. If we eat more local and organic food, most of us will consume fewer animal-source foods, which cannot be produced in large quantity and chemical-free in our neighborhoods. But livestock and meat raise such pressing concerns that they also need to be addressed directly and given priority in the food security movement and in public policy.

The evidence is overwhelming that we need to eat differently. It might seem we need to lower our expectations, but with environmentally healthy eating, we may ultimately be raising those expectations. We can expect big things of ourselves and our communities — that we learn, modify habits, work with citizen groups, press policymakers for change, and get involved in food. We can eat sustainably, healthfully, and compassionately, and help lower the stakes.

APPENDIX I

What's to Eat?
Tips and Recipes for Cutting the Meat

Making Meat-less Work

Learning to eat less meat can be an enjoyable project for the long term. It does require an adjustment in your habits and attitudes toward cooking and eating, but the ideas here can get you off to a strong start. Below are specific tips about the kinds of foods you can buy and how you make them into delicious meals. First, however, I've listed guidelines that help people transform their diets into meat-less ones. The beauty of these guidelines is that you can incorporate them gradually.

1. Make meat a side dish rather than the main attraction.

This can be as simple as serving only half your usual amount of meat, and then supplementing it with heartier helpings of potatoes, carrots, and green vegetables. Another adjustment that's almost as easy to make is to stop considering the meat item as your "main dish." Plant-based meals can be served tapas-style, with a number of small plates. Or, if you really like the idea of anchoring the meal with a main dish, try making it a vegetable dish or pasta. When you do include meat or fish in the meal, serve it as moderate portion on the side, not as the main focus of the meal.

2. Eat meatless at least one day a week.

One way to start this project is by joining Meatless Monday, the international movement discussed in Chapter 6. Go one day a week with no meat or seafood, or with no animal products at all. Consider going a step further and become a Weekday Vegetarian.[1]

3. In your favorite meals, substitute plant ingredients
for at least a portion of the animal ones.

It's not necessary to use vegetarian cookbooks, though many of them are beautiful, inspiring, and enjoyable. Many of your usual everyday meals can be made with few or no animal products. On pizza, minimize the salami and add extra tomatoes, peppers, mushrooms, and pitted olives. For stews, skip or limit the beef, and use root vegetables or a crumbled veggie burger patty, or chunks of tempeh (a fermented soybean product). If you like chili, make it as you normally would with kidney beans, tomatoes, herbs, and spices. But instead of ground beef, add just about any kind of bean (black, garbanzo, or pinto are good ones to try), vegetarian "ground round," small cubes of tofu, or extra tomatoes and kidney beans.

4. When eating out, explore vegetarian options
or ask for sustainable animal products.

At restaurants, look for menu items that do not include meat. If there are no veggie items, ask for something on the menu to be made without the animal products. Often, the kitchen can easily accommodate such requests. Sandwiches, wraps, and salads can all be made without meat. When eating out, for my main meal I sometimes order a couple of sides of vegetables and potatoes, all served on one plate. Sprinkle it with a teaspoon of olive oil, squeeze on some lemon, and it's an excellent meal.

Ask if they serve organic, or otherwise sustainable, animal products. Help restaurants join the movement by suggesting they offer eco-friendly animal products and more meatless meals. Don't be shy. You're the customer.

5. At home, prepare vegetables in much
the same ways as meat or seafood.

Vegetables like broccoli, carrots, and green beans can be sautéed, broiled, or barbequed with herbs and condiments similar to those you might use for chicken, beef, pork, or fish. Pan-seared spinach with garlic is one of my favorite food items. For oven cooking, rather than roast a large cut of meat, you can roast carrots, onions, parsnips, and fennel.

Oven-baked Brussels sprouts or potatoes are so crispy and sweet that people rave about them.

6. Experiment with new foods, recipes, and cuisines.

At the grocery store, occasionally pick up a vegetable you've never tasted before. Find a recipe for it, or just try steaming it. Most fresh foods need minimal assistance for flavor. Try dishes from cultures that minimize the meat. Some meals drawn from Italian, Mexican, Indian, and Chinese cuisines can be prepared in less than 30 minutes. Try making curried vegetables with garbanzo beans; pasta with tomato sauce; or tortillas with pinto beans, rice, and avocado. Look for ideas from restaurants, especially vegetarian ones. Vegetarian restaurants and cafés have proliferated not only in number, but also in the types of fare offered. They now range from casual to high-end fine dining, and from specific ethnicities to international cuisine. And if you can't actually eat at a particular restaurant, you can often find their menus online.[2]

Dishes to Try

This is not a cookbook, and I am not a chef. However, I love working with vegetables, grains, legumes, herbs, and spices in some of the infinite combinations possible. The following are basic and quick-to-prepare meals of the type we eat at home often. Nothing gourmet, just my family's kind of food.

First a few mentions, starting with flavor. Many people add interest to meals using salt and pepper or bottled sauces. Sauces are a venerable addition to food preparation, but I've stopped using thick store-bought varieties, which are often heavy with salt, sugar, and calories. Try to make your own light sauces and work toward meals that allow for the taste of the food itself to emerge. When I cook, I use a sprinkle of homemade vinaigrette on many different vegetable dishes. Olive oil and wine vinegar, or flax oil and lemon, are good combinations to start with.

Flavor is best achieved with a minimum of salt, since most of us already take in more sodium than is good for us these days. Try no-calorie herbs and spices instead. I decide what flavor I'd like for a dish, then choose accordingly. For Mediterranean tastes, I often use basil, oregano, and dill, along with some good olive oil. For Chinese tastes, I reach for ginger, tamari or soy sauce, and sesame oils. For Indian tastes, I use curry ingredients, including cumin and turmeric, and various vegetable oils. (Indian flavoring can seem complicated, but try experimenting with them and just see what you like.) For easy Mexican-style dishes, I like to use chili, garlic, onion, and cilantro and tomato salsas.

"Legumes" may sound unfamiliar, but the term mostly just refers to cooked beans. To explore this food group, set aside the notion that you need to spend time soaking and cooking beans. I use mostly pre-cooked and canned garbanzo, kidney, and white varieties. To start, buy a few cans and add a spoonful or two of different types to salads and other dishes. It's not difficult to find organic canned beans that have no additives. Introduce beans slowly to your diet to let your body get accustomed.

Our favorite carbohydrates are potatoes, pasta, brown or wild rice, buckwheat kasha, spelt, quinoa (pronounced "KEEN-wah"), or millet. You can add variety to your meals with the less familiar grains, some of which take only 20–30 minutes to make, unlike brown rice which takes closer to an hour. Any type of grain can be spiced up with onion or other small edibles, as in the pilaf recipe below. For pastas, experiment with different shapes and constituent grains along with the familiar semolina wheat. We enjoy kamut, spelt, and whole wheat pastas.

For the main meal of the day, we like to have a staple carb, plus one or two vegetable dishes, and some kind of legume. Here are two menus for evening meals from our kitchen. Feel free to mix and match with these recipes. Amounts serve 2–4 people, depending on their appetites and how many of the dishes you include.

Meal #1:
Cumin-Carrot Rice Pilaf
Sautéed Leafy Greens or Stir-Fried Vegetables
Tomato-Garlic Orange Lentils

■ Cumin-Carrot Rice Pilaf

For rice:
¾ cup brown rice, plus ¼ cup wild rice
2 cups water

For pilaf mixture:
½ cup finely chopped carrots
1–2 tablespoons chopped leeks or red onion
1 stalk chopped celery
1 teaspoon chopped garlic
2 teaspoons olive oil
1–1½ teaspoon cumin powder
1 teaspoon lemon zest or finely chopped lemon rind
juice of 1 fresh lemon
a little salt and pepper

Optional extras for color and variety: bits of green or red pepper, shelled green edamame soy beans, dried cranberries, chopped radishes, pumpkin seeds, or shaved almonds, and parsley for topping.

For the rice, add rice and water to a deep saucepan, bring to a boil then simmer for 45–60 minutes. For the pilaf, in a separate saucepan, add the main ingredients and sauté on medium heat until the onions, carrot bits, celery, and any other ingredients are soft. Stir in the cumin, lemon, and seasoning.

Pour rice into a serving dish, then scoop the pilaf mixture over and fold it throughout the rice. Add a topping of chopped parsley or such if you choose. Squeeze on more lemon, and serve.

■ Sautéed Leafy Greens

One favorite in our home is what we just call "greens" for the vast array of leafy plant tops available. Sautéed greens are amazing for taste, nutrition, and ease of preparation. This recipe suggests chard, but you can use kale or others. Hearty types like collards require a few extra minutes on the stove.

1 large bunch of green or multicolored chard
1 tablespoon olive oil
sprinkle of salt

Wash the greens and tear out the largest of the thick spines. Cut or tear the leaves and toss them into a saucepan with a splash of water. Drizzle a little olive oil and add a pinch of salt. Cook uncovered on medium heat for 5–10 minutes until the greens are soft. Boil or drain off any excess water. Slide the greens into a serving dish and squeeze on a small amount of fresh lemon or white wine vinegar. Serve with grains, or on toast, or as a simple side dish. Sigh. This is real food.

There are no fixed rules about specific ingredients here. To this dish we sometimes add finely chopped onion or thin peels of carrot for color. Sometimes I poach tomato slices atop the chard as it's cooking. When the greens are almost done, I add a sprinkle of balsamic vinegar over it all, and serve.

■ Stir-Fried Vegetables

Stir-fries come in endless varieties. What defines a stir-fry for me are its Asian flavors, quick cooking, and mix of good, basic vegetables. Recipe books will give you plenty of options, but here is one approach:

1 tablespoon oil (sesame or peanut, or something more neutral, like safflower oil)
¼ cup chopped onion
1 teaspoon chopped garlic
1 teaspoon chopped ginger
1–2 tablespoon soy sauce, tamari, or the like
1 cup chopped carrot
1–2 cups broccoli, rough-chopped or in florets

Optional: a handful of chopped vegetables such as cauliflower, white cabbage, red bell pepper, mushrooms, bok choy, snow peas, or almost any bean sprout.

In heavy pan on medium to high heat, add oil, onion, garlic, ginger, onion, carrot, and any other hardy vegetables. Sear briefly, add a splash of water, and cover to steam for a couple of minutes. Now add the softer vegetables, plus the tamari or soy. When the vegetables have softened a little, the stir-fry is ready to plate. I sometimes sprinkle a few sesame seeds on top, and serve beside brown rice or other grains.

Alternatively, I sometimes make a stir-fry that is mostly cabbage, a gorgeous vegetable that doesn't get much limelight but is substantial, delicious, and full of nutrients. Try the following ingredients, cut thinly by hand or chopped into bits in the food processor: 1 cup white cabbage, ¼ cup white or red onion. Optional: ¼ cup red cabbage, ¼ cup carrot. For this variation, I use less or lighter-colored soy sauces, so as not to discolor the cabbage.

■ Tomato-Garlic Orange Lentils

Lentils are wonderful food that can be included in soups and stews, or made into dishes like meatless meatloaf. We like lentils as a side dish. Quickest to cook are the yellow/orange variety, which we prepare as follows:

¼ cup dry orange/yellow lentils
1½–2 cups water
1 chopped tomato (or a few spoonfuls of canned diced tomato)
½ teaspoon chopped garlic
pinch of salt or other seasoning

Optionally, you can add any of: fine-chopped onion or cut spinach, or a little powdered cumin or curry.

Everything goes in at once. Bring it to a boil, then simmer until the lentils are soft, roughly 20 minutes, depending whether you'd prefer it light and liquid (in which case, cook it for less time) or rich and thick (in which case, keep simmering it to let more water boil off). If it's thin and soup-like, I serve individual portions in small bowls. If it is thicker, I spoon the lentils over potatoes or grains.

Meal #2:
Pasta with Tomato-Caper Sauce
Oven-Roasted Vegetables or Pan-Seared Garlic Spinach
Salad with Beans

■ Pasta with Tomato-Caper Sauce

We like varying the types and shapes of pasta we use, including short ones like penne and rotini as well as spaghetti, angel hair and other long varieties. Cooks all have their own pasta preferences, and many are sticklers for detail, but this quick sauce serves us well. The capers provide interest, and the rest is just a tasty tomato sauce. We try to keep the sauce fairly liquid, and not let it get thick or heavy. To keep it light, avoid using tomato paste, or use only small amounts of it.

For pasta:
1 cup dried pasta
3 cups boiling water

For sauce:
1 tablespoon olive oil
½ medium onion chopped fine
1 teaspoon chopped garlic
1 14-ounce can diced tomatoes (or 3 fresh, diced tomatoes)
1 tablespoon dried basil
2 tablespoons pickled capers
a little salt and pepper

Optional additions: pitted black olives, small-cubed eggplant, fine-chopped zucchini, chopped fresh basil, 1 teaspoon tomato paste.

Cook pasta in boiling water until it is softened, but still has body. In a separate saucepan, sauté onion and garlic for a few minutes, then add tomatoes and the rest of the ingredients. Simmer for 10–15 minutes. Once served, sprinkle on a little cheese if people wish.

■ Oven-Roasted Vegetables

What's not to love about carrots, Brussels sprouts, or potatoes done in the oven? Almost any full-bodied vegetable will do, including root vegetables like parsnips and turnips.

2 cups of trimmed vegetables in good-sized chunks
2 tablespoons olive oil
pinch of salt

Arrange chunks loosely in an ovenproof dish that has a tight-fitting lid. Drizzle with olive oil and sprinkle with salt. Cook covered for half an hour, in a 350–375 degree oven. Then remove the top of the baking dish in preparation for another half-hour in the oven. At this point you can add an optional ¼–½ cup chopped white or red onion, and/or 1 tablespoon chopped garlic. When the vegetables are crisp, serve hot.

You can faux-roast vegetables more quickly, on the stove, by boiling them for a few minutes until half-done, then sautéing them in a tablespoon or so of olive oil at medium heat for 5–10 minutes. Add a little garlic and onion around the sides and a small amount of salt and pepper. You can also add herbs and spices, such as dill, basil, or cumin. When doing potatoes (or summer squash, carrots or other veggies), make sure the knife-cut, or inside, faces are touching the pan, so they'll brown nicely. No need to turn them or fuss at all. Pry them off the pan with a flat spatula and serve.

■ Pan-Seared Garlic Spinach

This is a variation on the sautéed leafy greens above. The softness of spinach is heaven, as is the addition of garlic, which goes well with cooked spinach.

one bunch of spinach
1 teaspoon very finely chopped garlic
1 tablespoon olive oil
sprinkle of salt or other light seasoning

Heat a saucepan or frying pan to medium-high. Prepare the spinach by cutting away most of the stems, washing the leaves well, and cutting them once or twice, into large pieces. Place in the hot saucepan. No oil required yet; spinach sheds a large amount of water and will cook largely in its own liquid. Mix together the garlic and oil, and drizzle it on as the spinach is cooking. Add a tiny pinch of salt. In only a few moments, the spinach will have wilted and its water boiled off. Remove the spinach with a spatula or large spoon, and serve it immediately. Squeeze on a little lemon, if you like. You can use the spinach as a stuffing for tomatoes or other vegetables. But it's delicious as a simple side dish or served on warm grains.

■ Salad with Beans

I alternate between what I call "soft salads" based on lettuces, arugula, and other gentle ingredients, and "hard salads" based on heavier greens, such as kales and cabbage. Here is one of each.

Option #1: Kale Salad with Kidney Beans and Toasted Sesame Oil

For salad:

one bunch fresh curly green kale, with tough spines removed and the leaves cut into small pieces

½–1 cup of fine-chopped vegetables (e.g., red or white cabbage, round red radishes, or broccoli)

a few tablespoons of pre-cooked kidney or other dark-colored beans

For vinaigrette:

¼ cup toasted sesame oil

1 tablespoon white wine vinegar

1 tablespoon lemon juice

1 tablespoon tamari or soy sauce

a good pinch of ginger, either powdered or chopped

Put cut vegetables into a bowl, add vinaigrette, and toss thoroughly. Refrigerate for at least an hour before serving, to infuse the vegetables with the dressing and to soften the kale. This salad can be served for lunch or dinner with other dishes, or it can be plated over warm brown rice or other grains, as an Asian-inspired rice bowl.

Option #2: Mixed Greens, Herb, and White Bean Salad with Flax-Lemon Vinaigrette

Any delicate lettuces or greens will do, such as butter lettuce or
   arugula,
generous amounts of chopped fresh dill, mint, and/or parsley
   (as much as ¼ cup each),
a few tablespoons of cooked and drained white beans (cannellini,
   garbanzo, navy, lima, etc.)

For vinaigrette:
⅛ cup flax oil
juice of 1 lemon
tiny bit of salt and pepper
a drop of Dijon mustard, if desired

Nothing fancy here. Wash the greens, then tear them into the bowl and
add the rough-cut herbs and the beans. Whisk the vinaigrette ingredients together. Just moments before serving (not before, or everything
will get soggy) toss the salad with the vinaigrette.

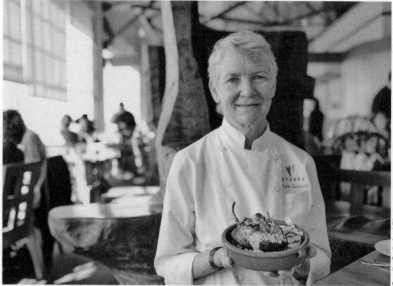

Credit: Seth Joel Photography

Annie Somerville of Greens restaurant in San Francisco.

Fire-Roasted Poblano Chilies
filled with Corn, Cheddar, and Cilantro

The smoky heat of poblano chilies makes them ideal for stuffing. At Greens, we grill them directly over an open flame until their skins blister and char, then let them steam in their own heat, so they're easy to peel. We season the corn filling with jalapenos, but you can also use serrano or other chilies instead. Serve with Fire-Roasted Salsa. This recipe serves 4.

4 poblano chilies, about 1 pound
½ tablespoon olive or vegetable oil
¼ large yellow onion, diced, about ½ cup
Salt and pepper
2 ears of corn, shaved, about 2 cups kernels
1 or 2 jalapeno chilies, seeded and diced
½ teaspoon chipotle puree
2 tablespoons coarsely chopped cilantro

1 teaspoon chopped fresh oregano or marjoram

1 teaspoon chopped fresh sage

3 ounces cheddar or smoked cheddar cheese, grated, about ¾ cup

Oil for the baking dish

Grill the chilies directly over the flame, using metal tongs to turn them until the skin is completely blistered and charred. Remove from the burner, transfer to a bowl, and cover; the chilies will steam as they cool.

Preheat the oven to 375° F. Heat the olive oil in a sauté pan and add the onions and a pinch each salt and pepper. Sauté over medium heat until the onions begin to soften, about 3 minutes. Add the corn, jalapenos, and ¼ cup water to keep the corn mixture from sticking to the pan. Cook over low heat until the corn is tender, about 5 minutes. Transfer to a bowl and set aside to cool.

Peel the chilies, carefully removing the skin around the stems as you go. Make a lengthwise slit in each chili and remove the seeds. Sprinkle lightly with salt and set them aside.

Lightly oil a baking dish. Season the corn mixture with the chipotle purée, herbs, cheese, ¼ teaspoon salt, and a pinch of pepper. Stuff each chili with ⅓ to ½ cup filling, depending on their size, being careful to keep the stems in place. The stuffed chilies should be firm, but not overly full. Place them seam-side up in the dish, cover and bake until the filling is heated through and the chilies are puffed, 25 to 30 minutes. Serve immediately.

Variation: If fresh oregano or marjoram and sage are not available, increase the chopped cilantro to ¼ cup.

Chipotle Puree

This fiery puree of smoked jalapeno chilies is indispensable in the Greens kitchen. We use canned chipotle chilies packed in adobo, a spicy sauce of the chilies, tomatoes, and vinegar. Puree a whole can at a time in a small food processor or blender and refrigerate in an airtight container. It keeps for weeks in the refrigerator. And you can freeze it too.

Fire-Roasted Salsa

*This rustic salsa has a taste that's smoky and rich. The plum tomatoes
are grilled over coals—their firm, dense flesh keeps the salsa from
being watery—and cilantro and lime juice keep the flavors bright.
This makes about 2 cups.*

1 pound plum tomatoes, cored
½ medium onion
1 or 2 jalapeno or serrano chilies
Olive oil
Salt and pepper
1½ to 2 tablespoons fresh lime juice
2 tablespoons coarsely chopped cilantro

Prepare the grill. Brush the tomato, onion, and chilies with olive oil
and sprinkle with salt and pepper. When the coals are ready, grill until
the tomatoes and chilies are soft and their skins are blistered and the
onion is grilled on all sides. Set aside to cool. Coarsely chop the onion
and tomatoes and toss in a bowl. Slice the chili in half lengthwise and
remove the stems and seeds. Chop the chili and toss with the tomato
mixture, along with 1½ tablespoons lime juice, ¼ teaspoon salt, and
a pinch of pepper. Season to taste with salt and lime juice, if needed.
Toss in the cilantro just before serving.

Resources: Research and Organizations to Know

The following lists give a taste of the fascinating work being conducted on the issues discussed in this book. You'll find expanded lists of resources on the website for this book.

Reports

CAFOs Uncovered: The Untold Costs of Confined Animal Feeding Operations. Doug Gurian-Sherman. Cambridge, MA: Union of Concerned Scientists, 2008.

Citizens' Guide to Confronting a Factory Farm. Beyond Factory Farming, 2007. citizensguide.ca.

Cool Farming: Climate Impacts of Agriculture and Mitigation Potential. J. Bellarby et al., Amsterdam: Greenpeace International, 2008.

Corporate Social Responsibility Summary Report 2010/11. Smithfield Foods, smith fieldcommitments.com.

Eating the Planet? How We Can Feed the World Without Trashing It. Friends of the Earth and Compassion in World Farming, 2009.

Embracing a Sustainable Future. Winnipeg: Manitoba Pork Council, 2011.

Factory Farm Nation: How American Turned Its Livestock Farms into Factories. Food and Water Watch, 2010. factoryfarmmap.org.

Food, Nutrition, Physical Activity, and the Prevention of Cancer: A Global Perspective. World Cancer Research Fund and American Institute for Cancer Research, 2007.

Happier Meals: Rethinking the Global Meat Industry. Danielle Nierenberg. World Watch Paper 171, 2005.

Healthy Planet Eating: How Lower Meat Diets can Save Lives and the Planet. Friends of the Earth. Oxford: Oxford University, 2010.

How Low Can We Go? An Assessment of Greenhouse Gas Emissions from the UK Food System and the Scope for Reduction by 2050. Eric Audsley et al., World Wildlife Fund UK and the Food Climate Research Network, 2010.

Livestock Consumption and Climate Change: A Framework for Dialogue Tom Mac-Millan and Rachael Durrant, Brighton, UK: Food Ethics Council and World Wildlife Fund, 2009.

Livestock's Long Shadow: Environmental Issues and Options. Henning Steinfeld, Pierre Gerber, Tom Wassenaar, Vincent Castel, Mauricio Rosales, and Cees de Haan, Rome: United Nations Food and Agriculture Organization, 2006.

Meat Eater's Guide to Climate Change and Health. Kari Hamerschlag, Washington: Environmental Working Group, 2011.

Putting Meat on the Table: Industrial Farm Animal Production in America. Pew Commission on Industrial Farm Animal Production, Baltimore, MD: Johns Hopkins Bloomberg School of Public Health, 2008.

Raising the Steaks: Global Warming and Pasture-Raised Beef Production in the U.S. Doug Gurian-Sherman. Cambridge, MA: Union of Concerned Scientists, 2011.

Slaughtering the Amazon. Amsterdam: Greenpeace International, 2009.

The Global Benefits of Eating Less Meat. Mark Gold. Compassion in World Farming. Hampshire, UK: CIWF, 2004.

Understanding Concentrated Animal Feeding Operations and Their Impact on Communities. Carrie Hribar. National Assn of Local Boards of Health, 2010.

Water for Food, Water for Life: A Comprehensive Assessment of Water Management in Agriculture. David Molden, ed., International Water Management Institute. London: Earthscan, 2007.

What's on Your Plate: The Hidden Costs of Industrial Animal Agriculture in Canada. World Society for the Protection of Animals (WSPA), Toronto: WSPA. 2012.

Why Livestock and Humane, Sustainable Agriculture Matter at Rio+20. WSPA International, 2012. wspa-international.org

World Livestock 2011: Livestock in Food Security. Rome: Food and Agriculture Organization, 2011.

Books

Bittman, Mark. *Food Matters: A Guide to Conscious Eating.* NY: Simon & Schuster, 2009.

Blatner, Dawn Jackson. *The Flexitarian Diet: The Mostly Vegetarian Way to Lose Weight, Be Healthier, Prevent Disease, and Add Years to Your Life.* NY: McGraw-Hill, 2009.

Blatt, Harvey. *America's Food: What You Don't Know About What You Eat.* Cambridge, MA: MIT Press, 2008.

Brubaker, Elizabeth. *Greener Pastures: Decentralizing the Regulation of Agricultural Pollution.* Toronto: University of Toronto Centre for Public Management Monograph Series, 2007.

Campbell, T. C. and Campbell, T. M. II. *The China Study: Startling Implications for Diet, Weight Loss and Long-Term Health.* Dallas: BenBella Books, 2006.

Cockrall-King, Jennifer. *Food and the City: Urban Agriculture and the New Food Revolution.* Amherst, NY: Prometheus Books, 2012.

D'Silva, Joyce and John Webster, eds. *The Meat Crisis: Developing More Sustainable Production and Consumption.* London: Earthscan, 2010.

Ervin, Alexander et al. *Beyond Factory Farming: Corporate Hog Barns and the Threat to Public Health, the Environment and Rural Communities.* Saskatoon: Canadian Centre for Policy Alternatives, 2003.

Fairlie, Simon. *Meat: A Benign Extravagance*. Hampshire: Permanent Publications, 2010.

Fearnley-Whittingstall, Jane. *The Ministry of Food: Thrifty Wartime Ways to Feed Your Family Today*. London: Hodder & Stoughton and the Imperial War Museum, 2010.

Foer, Jonathan Safran. *Eating Animals*. NY: Little, Brown, 2009.

Halweil, Brian. *Eat Here: Reclaiming Homegrown Pleasures in a Global Supermarket*. NY: Norton, 2004.

Imhoff, Daniel. *Food Fight: The Citizens' Guide to the Next Food and Farm Bill*. Healdsburg, CA: Watershed Media, 2012.

Imhoff, Daniel, ed., *The CAFO Reader: The Tragedy of Industrial Animal Factories*. Healdsburg, CA: Watershed Media, 2010.

Kimbrell, Andrew, ed., *The Fatal Harvest Reader: The Tragedy of Industrial Agriculture*. Washington D.C.: Island Press, 2002.

Kirby, David. *Animal Factory: The Looming Threat of Industrial Pig, Dairy, and Poultry Farms to Humans and the Environment*. NY: St. Martin's Press, 2010.

Ladner, Peter. *The Urban Food Revolution: Changing the Way We Feed Cities*. Gabriola Island, BC: New Society Publishers, 2011.

Lang, Tim, David Barling and Martin Caraher. *Food Policy: Integrating Health, Environment and Society*. Oxford University Press, 2009.

Lappe, Anna. *Diet for a Hot Planet: The Climate Crisis at the End of Your Fork and What You Can Do About It*. NY: Bloomsbury, 2010.

McKibben, Bill. *Eaarth: Making a Life on a Tough New Planet*. NY: St. Martin's Griffin, 2010.

McWilliams, James. *Just Food: Where Locavores Get It Wrong and How We Can Truly Eat Responsibly*. NY: Little, Brown, 2009.

Millstone, Eric and Tim Lang. *The Atlas of Food: Who Eats What, Where, and Why*. Berkeley: University of California Press, 2008.

Nestle, Marion. *What to Eat: An Aisle-by-Aisle Guide to Savvy Food Choices and Good Eating*. NY: North Point Press, 2006.

Nestle, Marion. *Food Politics: How the Food Industry Influences Nutrition and Health*. Berkeley: University of California Press, 2003.

Niman, Nicolette Hahn. *Righteous Porkchop: Finding a Life and Good Food Beyond Factory Farms*. NY: Harper, 2010.

Patel, Raj. *Stuffed and Starved: The Hidden Battle for the World Food System*. Brooklyn, NY: Melville House, 2007.

Pollan, Michael. *In Defense of Food: An Eater's Manifesto*. NY: Penguin, 2008.

Popkin, Barry. *The World is Fat: The Fads, Trends, Policies and Products That Are Fattening the Human Race*. NY: Avery, 2009.

Rayner, Geof and Tim Lang. *Ecological Public Health: Reshaping the Conditions for Good Health*. Abingdon: Earthscan/Routledge, 2012.

Roberts, Wayne. *The No-Nonsense Guide to World Food*. Oxford: New Internationalist, 2008.

Salatin, Joel. *Folks, This Ain't Normal: A Farmer's Advice for Happier Hens, Healthier People, and a Better World*. Center Street Publishers, 2011.

Steinfeld, Henning et al. *Livestock in a Changing Landscape: Drivers, Consequences and Responses,* Vol. I, Washington, D.C.: Island Press, 2010.
Suzuki, David. *The Sacred Balance: Rediscovering Our Place in Nature.* Vancouver: Greystone Books, 1997.
Weis, Tony. *The Global Food Economy: The Battle for the Future of Farming.* London: Zed Books, 2007.

Articles

Burkholder, JoAnn et al. "Impacts of waste from concentrated animal feeding operations on water quality," *Env Health Perspec* 115(2) 308–312, Feb 2007.
De Bakker, Erik, and Hans Dagevos. "Reducing meat consumption in today's consumer society: Questioning the citizen-consumer gap," *J Agric Enviro Ethics* Sept 2011.
Cross, A. J. et al. "A prospective study of red and processed meat intake in relation to cancer risk." *PLoS Med* 4(12) Dec 2007.
Garnett, Tara. "Livestock-related greenhouse gas emissions: Impacts and options for policy makers," *Environmental Science and Policy* 12: 491–503, 2009.
Friel, Sharon et al. "Public health benefits of strategies to reduce greenhouse gas emissions: Food and agriculture." *The Lancet* Nov 25, 2009.
MacRae, Rod. "A joined-up food policy for Canada," *J Hunger Environmental Nutrition* 6(4) 424–457, 2011.
McMichael, Anthony, John Powles, Colin Butler, and Ricardo Uauy. "Food, livestock production, energy, climate change and health," *The Lancet* 370(9594) 1253–1263, 2007.
Mooney, Harold. "Consequences of livestock production: Environmental, health, and social consequences of livestock production," p. 67–68. In Steinfeld et al., *Livestock in a Changing Landscape: Drivers, Consequences and Responses,* Vol. I, Washington, D.C.: Island Press, 2010.
Naylor, Rosamond et al. "Losing the links between livestock and land," *Science* 310 1621–1622, 2005.
Nestle, Marion. "Big food, big agra, and the research university," *Academe* Nov–Dec 2010, p. 47–49.
Pimentel, David and Marcia Pimentel. "Sustainability of meat-based and plant-based diets and the environment," *Am J Clin Nutr* 78: 660S–663S, 2003.
Pitesky, M., K. Stackhouse, and F. Mitloehner. "Clearing the air: Livestock's contribution to climate change," *Advances in Agronomy* 103: 1–40, 2009.
Popkin, Barry. "Reducing meat consumption has multiple benefits for the world's health," *Arch Intern Med* 169(6) 543–545, Mar 23, 2009.
Sapkota, A. R., L. Y. Lefferts, S. McKenzie, and P. Walker. "What do we feed to food-production animals? A review of animal feed ingredients and their potential impacts on human health," *Env Health Perspec* 115: 663–670, 2007.
Schreier, Hans. "Agricultural water policy challenges in B.C.," *Policy Options* Jul–Aug 2009.
Silbergeld, Ellen, Jay Graham, and Lance Price. "Industrial food animal produc-

tion, antimicrobial resistance, and human health," *Ann Rev Public Health* 29: 151–169, 2008.

Walker, Polly et al. "Public health implications of meat production and consumption," *Public Health Nutrition* 8(4) 348–356, 2005.

Weber, Christopher and H. Scott Matthews. "Food-miles and the relative climate impacts of food choices in the United States," *Enviro Sci and Tech* 42: 3508–3513, 2008.

Organizations and Institutes

Beyond Factory Farming — beyondfactoryfarming.org
Promotes socially responsible livestock production. Based in Saskatoon, Saskatchewan.

Center for a Livable Future — jhsph.edu/clf
Based at the Johns Hopkins Bloomberg School of Public Health, Baltimore, MD. Researches interconnections among diet, food, health, and the environment.

EarthSave International — earthsave.org; earthsave.ca
California-based group promoting plant-based diets. Also see Earthsave Canada, a Vancouver-based group educating people on consequences of food choices.

Farm Forward — farmforward.com
Located in Portland, Oregon, promotes conscientious food choices, better treatment of farm animals, and sustainable agriculture.

Farm Sanctuary — farmsanctuary.org
Headquartered in Watkins Glen, NY. Works to protect animals and promote compassionate living.

Food and Water Watch — foodandwaterwatch.org
Washington-based organization for safe, clean and sustainable food, water, and fish.

Humane Society of the United States — humanesociety.org
Based in Washington, this multifaceted organization is the largest US animal protection group.

Keep Antibiotics Working — keepantibioticsworking.com
Chicago-based coalition of groups aiming to protect antibiotics from overuse, especially in food animals.

Pew Commission on Industrial Farm Animal Production — ncifap.org
Baltimore, MD: Johns Hopkins Bloomberg School of Public Health.

Physicians' Committee for Responsible Medicine — pcrm.org
Washington-based organization promoting healthy plant-based eating and preventive medicine.

Socially Responsible Agricultural Project — sraproject.org
Idaho-based organization for sustainable livestock and food production.

Sustainable Table — sustainabletable.org
New York-based educational organization aiming to "educate, advocate, cultivate" for local and sustainable food.

Union of Concerned Scientists — ucsusa.org/food_and_agriculture
Washington-based group working on issues including ecologically viable agriculture.

Vancouver Humane Society — vancouverhumanesociety.bc.ca
Promotes animal welfare, including for farm animals. Also see other local and national humane societies.

Waterkeeper Alliance — waterkeeper.org
Advocacy organization based in New York, engaged in hands-on water protection in the United States, Canada, and internationally.

World Society for the Protection of Animals — wspa-usa.org, wspa.ca
International organization for animal welfare, including in food production.

Notes

Introduction

1. Henning Steinfeld et al., *Livestock's Long Shadow: Environmental Issues and Options*. Rome: United Nations Food and Agriculture Organization (FAO), 2006; Joyce D'Silva and John Webster, eds., *The Meat Crisis: Developing More Sustainable Production and Consumption*. London: Earthscan, 2010; Daniel Imhoff, ed., *The CAFO Reader: The Tragedy of Industrial Animal Factories*. Watershed Media, 2010; Carrie Hribar, *Understanding Concentrated Animal Feeding Operations and Their Impact on Communities*. Bowling Green, Iowa: National Assn of Local Boards of Health, 2010; World Society for the Protection of Animals, *What's on Your Plate? The Hidden Costs of Industrial Animal Agriculture in Canada*. Toronto, 2012.

2. Polly Walker et al., "Public Health Implications of Meat Production and Consumption," *Public Health Nutrition* 8(4) 348–356, 2005; *Putting Meat on the Table: Industrial Farm Animal Production in America*. Pew Commission on Industrial Farm Animal Production, Baltimore, MD: Johns Hopkins Bloomberg School of Public Health, 2008.

3. D'Silva and Webster, eds., *The Meat Crisis*. 2010.

4. Joyce D'Silva is director of public affairs and former chief executive of Compassion in World Farming (CIWF), a leading European non-governmental organization for farm animal welfare. E-mail to the author, Dec 2, 2011; This is supported by findings in "Eating the Planet: How We Can Feed the World Without Trashing It," CIWF and Friends of the Earth, 2009.

5. I have worked as a UNESCO consultant in West Africa training journalists and have traveled in many other developing and industrialized regions.

6. Tim Lang, Michelle Wu, and Martin Caraher, "Meat and Policy: Charting a Course through the Complexity," in D'Silva and Webster, *The Meat Crisis*, 2010, p. 255. Dr. Lang heads the Centre for Food Policy at City University in London, England. I studied with Dr. Lang along with Drs. David Barling and Martin Caraher to earn an MSc in Food Policy.

7. Steinfeld et al., *Livestock's Long Shadow*. 2006, p. xxiv.

8. T. Colin Campbell and Thomas Campbell II, co-authors of *The China Study* (Dallas: BenBella Books, 2006) argue that meat undermines health, and that, rather than cut back, it is easier for consumers to go "all the way" to a completely plant-based diet, p. 244.

9. I had asked during question period whether consumers shouldn't consider decreasing their meat intake.

10. Maybe I should stop bringing along my slide presentations.

11. Don Webb, personal interview with the author in N. Carolina, August 2011. (Chitlins are hog intestines, a key ingredient in several dishes popular in the American South.)

12. John Robbins, *Diet for a New America*. Tiburon, CA: Kramer, 1987.

13. Barry Popkin, "Reducing Meat Consumption Has Multiple Benefits for the World's Health," *Arch Intern Med* 169(6) 545, Mar 23, 2009.

Chapter 1

1. UN Food and Agriculture Organization (FAO) publications and statistics from e-mail communication with staff of Livestock Information, Sector Analysis and Policy Branch, FAO.

2. Gowri Koneswaran and Danielle Nierenberg, "Global Farm Animal Production and Global Warming: Impacting and Mitigating Climate Change," *Env Health Perspec* 116(5) 2008.

3. Christopher Delgado et al., *Livestock to 2020: The Next Food Revolution*. IFPRI/FAO/ILRI, 1999.

4. Steinfeld et al., *Livestock's Long Shadow*. 2006, p. xx.

5. Shayle Shagam, livestock and poultry analyst, USDA, e-mail to author, January 2012; Also, USDA statistical tables, ers.usda.gov, 2012; Mark Bittman, "We're Eating Less Meat. Why?" Opinionator, *New York Times*, Jan 10, 2012.

6. Mark Bittman, "We're Eating Less Meat," 2012.

7. "StatsCan Food Statistics 2009," *Statistics Canada*, 2010; USDA Economic Research Service, ers.usda.gov, 2011.

8. *World Livestock 2011: Livestock in Food Security*. UN FAO, Rome, 2011; Anthony McMichael et al., "Food, Livestock Production, Energy, Climate Change and Health," *The Lancet* 370(9594) 1253–1263, 2007.

9. C. R. Daniel et al., "Trends in Meat Consumption in the United States," *Public Health Nutrition* 14(4) 575–583, 2011; McMichael et al., 2007; USDA Agriculture Fact Book, "Profiling Food Consumption in America, 2001–2002." Some scientists say Americans eat much more than 200 pounds/year. See Pimentel and Pimentel, "Sustainability of Meat-Based and Plant-Based Diets and the Environment," *Am J Clin Nutr* 78:3 (suppl) 660S–663S, 2003.

10. *USDA Agriculture Fact Book*. 2001–2002, p. 14. Per capita, the top ten meat-eating countries in the world, in order, are Uruguay, the United States, Cyprus, Spain, Denmark, New Zealand, Australia, Canada, France, and Ireland, according to Andrew Speedy, in "Global Production and Consumption of Animal Source Foods," *J of Nutrition* 2003.

11. McMichael et al., 2007.

12. Steinfeld et al., 2006, p. xx. Global meat production is projected to go from 229 million tons in 2000 to 465 million tons in 2050.

13. Anthony McMichael and Ainslie Butler, "Environmentally Sustainable and Equitable Meat Consumption in a Climate Change World," p. 173–189, in D'Silva and Webster, eds., *The Meat Crisis: Developing More Sustainable Production and Consumption.* 2010, p. 173.

14. Barry Popkin, *The World Is Fat: The Fads, Trends, Policies, and Products That Are Fattening the Human Race.* NY: Avery, 2009, p. 17–18.

15. Anthony McMichael, *Planetary Overload: Global Environmental Change and the Health of the Human Species.* Cambridge University Press, 1995, p. 92.

16. Brian Halweil and Danielle Nierenberg, "Meat and Seafood: The Global Diet's Most Costly Ingredients," p. 61–74, in *State of the World 2008.* Worldwatch Institute, NY: Norton, p. 61.

17. Adam Drewnowski and Barry Popkin, "The Nutrition Transition: New Trends in the Global Diet," *Nutrition Reviews* 55(2) 1997.

18. Manitoba Pork Council, *Embracing a Sustainable Future.* 2011, p. 22.

19. "Diet, Nutrition and the Prevention of Chronic Diseases," World Health Organization Technical Report Series 916, Geneva: WHO, 2003.

20. Steinfeld et al., 2006, p. 275.

21. Ibid., p. xx. Global milk production is expected to rise from 580 million tons in 2000 to 1,043 million tons by 2050.

22. The unsustainability of current fishing and seafood consumption has been widely documented. See Villy Christensen et al., "Fish Biomass in the World Ocean: A Century of Decline," Working Paper #2011–06, Fisheries Centre, University of B.C., 2011; David Jenkins et al., "Are Dietary Recommendations for the Use of Fish Oils Sustainable?" *Canad Med Assn Journal* 180(6), Mar 17, 2009; Bryan Walsh, "The End of the Line, *Time Magazine,* Jul 18, 2011.

23. "Increased Protection Urgently Needed for Tunas," International Union for the Conservation of Nature, Jul 7, 2011, iucn.org; "More Than Half of Tuna Species at Risk of Extinction, Say Conservationists," Press Assn., Jul 7, 2011. guardian.co.uk.

24. G. A. Rose, "Fisheries Resource and Science in Newfoundland and Labrador: An Independent Assessment," 2003, gov.nl.ca; Mark Kurlansky, *Cod: A Biography of the Fish That Changed the World.* Penguin, 1997; Paul Greenberg, *Four Fish: The Future of the Last Wild Food.* Penguin, 2010.

25. *Putting Meat on the Table: Industrial Farm Animal Production in America.* Pew Commission, 2008, p. 3.

26. "Terminology: CAFOs and Large Livestock Operations," USDA, nrcs.usda .gov.

27. Bernard Rollin, "Farm Factories: The End of Animal Husbandry," in Daniel Imhoff, ed., *The CAFO Reader.* Watershed Media, 2010, p. 6.

28. Joel Salatin, *Folks, This Ain't Normal: A Farmer's Advice for Happier Hens, Healthier People, and a Better World.* NY: Center Street Publishers, 2011.

29. Rosamond Naylor et al., "Losing the Links Between Livestock and Land," *Science* 10(310) 1621–1622, 2005.

30. David Kirby, *Animal Factory: The Looming Threat of Industrial Pig, Dairy, and Poultry Farms to Humans and the Environment*. St. Martin's Press, 2010, p. xiv.

31. Doug Gurian-Sherman, *CAFOs Uncovered: The Untold Costs of Confined Animal Feeding Operations*. Washington: Union of Concerned Scientists, 2008, p. 10.

32. *Factory Farm Nation: How America Turned Its Livestock Farms into Factories*. Food and Water Watch, 2010, factoryfarmmap.org, p. 2 and 19. These points are supported in other reports including the Pew Commission's *Putting Meat on the Table*, 2008.

33. Economists and scientists have documented government financial support for industrial livestock systems and its consequences, including lower retail prices for animal products. See the 2008 Pew Commission report *Putting Meat on the Table* and Harwood Schaffer et al., "Economics of Industrial Farm Animal Production," a Pew Report, 2008.

34. Gurian-Sherman, *CAFOs Uncovered*. 2008, p. 18–19.

35. Sustainable Table, "Animal Welfare," sustainabletable.org, accessed Jan 3, 2012; Mark Bittman, "Some Animals Are More Equal Than Others," Opinionator, *New York Times*, Mar 15, 2011.

36. "Hiding the Truth About Factory Farms," opinion pages, *New York Times*, Apr 26, 2011.

37. There is a large literature on these laws. For a legal summary, see Rebecca Turano, *Agricultural Disparagement Statutes: An Overview*. 2010, law .psu.edu.

38. However, an increasing interest in simple fare is reflected in publications including *Cucina Povera: Tuscan Peasant Cooking* by Pamela S. Johns (Andrews McMeel: Kansas City, Missouri, 2011).

39. Christopher Delgado et al., *Livestock to 2020: The Next Food Revolution*. IFPRI, 1999; Steinfeld et al., 2006.

40. Meat producers and retailers spend millions of dollars a year on advertising and marketing, as will be discussed in Ch. 9. Also see Gary Brester and Ted Schroeder, "The Impacts of Brand and Generic Advertising on Meat Demand," *Amer J Agr Econ* 77, Nov 1995, p. 969–979.

41. Rajendra K. Pachauri, foreword to *The Meat Crisis: Developing More Sustainable Production and Consumption*. D'Silva and Webster, eds., p. xvii. 2010. Dr. Pachauri is chair of the Intergovernmental Panel on Climate Change and was a recipient in 2007 of the Nobel Peace Prize.

42. Marion Nestle, *What to Eat: An Aisle-by-Aisle Guide to Savvy Food Choices and Good Eating*. NY: North Point Press, 2006, p. 140.

43. Tim Lang, David Barling and Martin Caraher, *Food Policy: Integrating Health, Environment and Society*. Oxford University Press, 2009, p. 27–8.

44. John Steinbeck, *The Grapes of Wrath*. Viking, 1939. This Pulitzer Prize-winning novel tells of the poor Joad family, victimized by Depression drought and hardship, who journeyed from Oklahoma to California for what they hoped would be a better life.

Chapter 2

1. Tara Garnett, "Livestock and Climate Change," in D'Silva and Webster, *The Meat Crisis*. 2010, p. 34.
2. Henning Steinfeld, et al., *Livestock's Long Shadow: Environmental Issues and Options*. Rome: UN FAO, 2006, p. xxi.
3. Steinfeld et al., 2006, p. xxi; Many other authors have also commented on the heavy use of land for livestock, e.g., Foley et al., "Solutions for a Cultivated Planet," *Nature* 478, Oct 2011, p. 337–342.
4. Steinfeld et al., 2006; Tara Garnett, "Livestock-Related Greenhouse Gas Emissions: Impacts and Options for Policy Makers," *Env Sci Policy* 12: 491–503, 2009.
5. Jennifer Jacquet et al., "Conserving Wild Fish in a Sea of Market-Based Efforts," *Oryx*, 2009, p. 53; Jacqueline Alder, et al., "Forage Fish: From Ecosystems to Markets," *Ann Rev Env Res* 33: 53–66, 2008.
6. David Pimentel and Marcia Pimentel, "Sustainability of Meat-Based and Plant-Based Diets and the Environment," *Amer J Clin Nutrition* 2003, p. 660S–663S.
7. Pimentel and Pimentel, 2003, p. 661S.
8. The term "ecological footprint" is now commonly heard, but credit for coining the term should go to Professor Bill Rees and graduate student Mathis Wackernagel from the University of B.C. They are the authors of *Our Ecological Footprint: Reducing Human Impact on the Earth*. Gabriola Island, B.C.: New Society Publishers, 1996.
9. Steinfeld et al., 2006.
10. Henning Steinfeld and Pierre Gerber, "Livestock Production and the Global Environment: Consume Less or Produce Better?" *PNAS* 107(43) Oct 26, 2010. Dr. Steinfeld also presented "Sustainable Protein Supply" at a European conference in March 2012, outlining potential efficiency gains that could accommodate demand for animal products.
11. Steinfeld et al., 2006, p. xxi.
12. Ibid., p. xx.
13. Ibid., p. xxi.
14. Several industry sources have made this claim about *Livestock's Long Shadow*. For example, the BeefSite e-publication, on Feb 1, 2012, said: "In 2006, the FAO concluded that livestock production was responsible for 18% of global greenhouse gas (GHG) emissions, and despite later admitting this figure was invalid, the number has stuck." I double-checked with the FAO authors, who confirmed that they never retracted the 18% figure.
15. Anthony McMichael et al., "Food, Livestock Production, Energy, Climate Change and Health," *The Lancet* 2007, p. 9. I'll say much more on this important article later in the book.
16. "Who Says Beef Production Isn't Sustainable?" The BeefSite, Feb 1, 2012, thebeefsite.com.
17. Steinfeld et al., 2006, p. xxi.

18. Christopher Matthews, Media Relations Officer, FAO, confirmed this for me in an e-mail, as did co-author Pierre Gerber. Said Mr. Matthews: "You're perfectly right. FAO has admitted that the comparison with transport was flawed (the livestock CO_2 emissions included deforestation and land-use change, while transport didn't include the manufacturing process or the raw materials, so it was a case of apples and pears). But we stand by the 18% and have never said it is invalid."

19. For example, see Dr. Judith Capper of Washington State University, wsu .academia.edu/JudeCapper. See also Greg Henderson, "Livestock's Long Shadow?" Drovers Cattle Network: American's Beef Business Source, Oct 16, 2007. Others who argue for meat production and consumption include Simon Fairlie in *Meat: A Benign Extravagance*. Chelsea Green, 2010.

20. American Meat Institute, meatami.com; sustainablemeatindustry.org, accessed Mar 3, 2012.

21. "Editorial: Who Says Beef Production Isn't Sustainable?" The BeefSite, weekly global cattle industry review, Feb 1, 2012. newsletters@5mpublishing.com. The newsletter quotes Dr. Judith Capper of Washington State University, who conducts research in livestock and sustainability.

22. Pitesky et al., 2009.

23. Robert Goodland and Jeff Anhang, "Livestock and Climate Change: What If the Key Actors in Climate Change Are Cows, Pigs and Chickens?" *World-Watch*, Nov/Dec 2009.

24. McMichael et al., 2007; D'Silva and Webster, 2010; Garnett, 2009; Halweil and Nierenberg, 2008.

25. Nicholas Stern, *The Economics of Climate Change: The Stern Review*. Cambridge University Press, 2007; Intergovernmental Panel on Climate Change (IPCC), *Climate Change 2007: The Physical Science Basis, Summary for Policymakers*.

26. IPCC, *Climate Change 2007: The Physical Science Basis*, p. 10.

27. IPCC, 2007, p. 115.

28. IPCC, ipcc.ch.

29. Steinfeld et al., 2006, p. 112; EPA, "Inventory of U.S. GHG Emissions and Sinks: 1990–2008," 2010; Bellarby et al., "Cool Farming: Climate Impacts of Agriculture and Mitigation Potential," 2008. This report says agriculture is responsible for 17–32% of all global human-induced GHG emissions and that livestock are directly or indirectly responsible for most of those agricultural emissions. See p. 5.

30. Greenpeace, "Slaughtering the Amazon," 2009, p. 1.

31. Steinfeld et al., 2006, p. xxiii.

32. Ibid., p. 43.

33. Ibid.

34. IPCC, "Land, Land-Use Change, and Forestry," ipcc.ch; FAO, "Incentives to Curb Deforestation Needed to Counter Climate Change. Two Billion Tonnes of Carbon Enter Atmosphere Each Year Due to Forest Loss," FAO Newsroom, Dec 2005, fao.org.

35. Biomass is the total of material from living (or recently living) plants or animals in a given environmental area. Biomass is packed with carbon and stored energy.
36. IPCC, 2007. The global warming potential (GWP) of methane (25–72 times as great as CO_2) depends on the time frame measured.
37. IPCC, 2007; Steinfeld et al., 2006.
38. Steinfeld, et al., 2006, p. 95, 96.
39. Ibid., p. 97.
40. Steinfeld et al., 2006, p. 112; Bellarby et al., 2008, p. 8.
41. Steinfeld, et al., 2006, p. 104–106.
42. Bellarby et al., 2008, p. 6; Simon Donner, "Surf or Turf: A Shift from Feed to Food Cultivation Could Reduce Nutrient Flux to the Gulf of Mexico," *Global Enviro Change* 17, 2007, p. 105–113.
43. Donner (2007) says 70% of grains from the Mississippi Basin go to livestock.
44. Steinfeld et al., 2006, p. 271, Table 7.1.
45. Christopher Weber and H. Scott Matthews, "Food-Miles and the Relative Climate Impacts of Food Choices in the United States," *Env Sci and Tech* 42: 3508–3513, 2008; Steinfeld et al., 2006; Garnett, 2010.
46. "Greenhouse Gas Emissions from the Dairy Sector: A Life Cycle Assessment," FAO Animal Production and Health Division, 2010, p. 11.
47. Weber and Matthews, 2008, p. 3508.
48. These numbers can vary dramatically in actual production systems and depending how they're calculated. To make 1 kg (2 pounds) of food, broiler chickens require about 2 kg (4.4 pounds) of feed, swine 5–6 kg of feed (11–13.2 pounds), and beef 13–30 kg (28.6–66 pounds) of grain or pasture forage, and milk cows require almost 1 kg of feed, according to Jessica Bellarby et al., "Cool Farming: Climate Impacts of Agriculture and Mitigation Potential," Greenpeace, 2008, p. 36.
49. Steinfeld et al., 2006, Tables 3.7–3.8, p. 97–99.
50. Weber and Matthews, 2008, p. 3511; Kari Hamerschlag, *Meat Eater's Guide to Climate Change and Health.* Environmental Working Group, 2011, ewg.org.
51. Elke Stehfest et al., "Climate Benefits of Changing Diet," *Climatic Change* 95: 83–102, 2009; Eric Audsley et al., *How Low Can We Go? An Assessment of Greenhouse Gas Emissions from the UK Food System and the Scope for Reduction by 2050.* Cranfield University, WWF and FCRN, 2009/2010.
52. Weber and Matthews, 2008, p. 3508.
53. Jessica Bellarby et al., "Cool Farming: Climate Impacts of Agriculture and Mitigation Potential," Greenpeace, 2008.
54. Environmental Working Group, *Meat Eaters' Guide.* 2011, p. 5.
55. X. P. C. Verge et al., "Long-Term Trends in Greenhouse Gas Emissions from the Canadian Poultry Industry," *J Applied Poultry Res* 18: 210–222, 2009; Environmental Working Group, *Meat Eater's Guide.* 2011.
56. Doug Gurian-Sherman, *Raising the Steaks: Global Warming and Pasture-Raised Beef Production in the U.S.* Union of Concerned Scientists, 2011, p. 3.

57. Eric Audsley et al., *How Low Can We Go? An Assessment of the Greenhouse Gas Emissions from the UK Food System and the Scope for Reduction by 2050*. Cranfield University, Jan 2010; Tara Garnett, *Cooking Up a Storm: Food, Greenhouse Gas Emissions and Our Changing Climate*. Food Climate Research Network, Surrey, UK, 2008; Weber and Matthews, 2008.
58. M. Berners-Lee et al., "The Relative Greenhouse Gas Impacts of Realistic Dietary Choices," *Energy Policy* 43: 184–190, Apr 2012.
59. Pitesky et al., 2009.
60. Audsley et al., 2010, p. 6.
61. Leo Horrigan, Robert Lawrence, and Polly Walker, "How Sustainable Agriculture Can Address the Environmental and Health Harms of Industrial Agriculture," *Env Health Perspec* 110(5) 454, 2002.
62. Steinfeld et al., 2006, p. 52.
63. Ibid., p. 222.
64. Ibid., p. 221–263.
65. Pro-Poor Livestock Policy Initiative, UN FAO, fao.org.
66. *World Livestock 2011: Livestock in Food Security*. UN FAO, Rome, 2011, p. 74.
67. McMichael et al., 2007.
68. Vision for Fair Food and Farming, visionforfairfood.org, Mar 4, 2012.
69. Audsley et al., 2009; Pete Smith et al., "Greenhouse Gas Mitigation in Agriculture," *Phil Trans R Soc B* 363: 789–813, 2008; Tom MacMillan and Rachael Durrant, *Livestock Consumption and Climate Change: A Framework for Dialogue*. London: Food Ethics Council and WWF, 2009; Stehfest et al., 2009; D'Silva and Webster, 2010.

Chapter 3

1. Waterkeeper Alliance is a New York-based organization, headed by environmental attorney Robert F. Kennedy, Jr., which directly patrols and protects waterways in the United States and other countries. As of late 2011, Larry Baldwin is no longer a Neuse Riverkeeper but is performing similar work as a CAFO contractor in North Carolina with Waterkeeper Alliance.
2. Biologist and Neuse expert Dr. JoAnn Burkholder estimates that more than a billion fish have died in the past few decades, while some environmentalists suggest the figure may be even higher.
3. Researchers including Dr. Burkholder say the fish were killed by toxins from the microorganism *Pfiesteria*. For another viewpoint, see J. P. Berry et al., "Are *Pfiesteria* Species Toxicogenic? Evidence Against Production of Ichthyotoxins by *Pfiesteria shumwayae*," *PNAS* 99(17) 2002.
4. North Carolina Riverkeepers and Waterkeeper Alliance, riverlaw.us; Howard Glasgow et al., "Field Ecology of Toxic Pfiesteria Complex Species and a Conservative Analysis of Their Role in Estuarine Fish Kills," *Env Health Perspec* 109(5) 2001; "What You Should Know About Pfiesteria and North Carolina's Waters," NC Dept of Environment and Natural Resources, enr.state.nc.us; JoAnn Burkholder et al., "Impacts of Waste from Concentrated Animal

Feeding Operations on Water Quality," *Env Health Perspec* 115(2) 308–312, Feb 2007; Meghan Rothenberger et al., "Long-Term Effects of Changing Land-Use Practices on Surface Water Quality in a Coastal River and Lagoonal Estuary," *Env Management* 44: 505–523, 2009; NC Dept of Environment and Natural Resources; U.S. Dept of Agriculture, portal.ncdenr.org.

5. James Barker, "Lagoon Design and Management for Livestock Waste Treatment and Storage," NC Cooperative Extension Service, 1996, bae.ncsu.edu.

6. Even the industry says lagoons have limited useful lifespans. See the National Hog Farmer website, nationalhogfarmer.com.

7. Dr. JoAnn Burkholder, William Neal Reynolds Distinguished Professor, Department of Plant Biology and Director, Center for Applied Aquatic Ecology, North Carolina State University, e-mail to author, July 21, 2011.

8. Smithfield Foods, videos on pork production and environmental management, murphybrownllc.com.

9. Dr. JoAnn Burkholder, e-mail to author, July 21, 2011.

10. JoAnn Burkholder et al., "Comprehensive Trend Analysis of Nutrients and Related Variables in a Large Eutrophic Estuary," *Limnol Oceanogr* 51(1, pt 2) 463–487, 2006; Meghan Rothenberger, JoAnn Burkholder, and Cavell Brownie, "Long-Term Effects of Changing Land-Use Practices on Surface Water Quality in a Coastal River and Lagoonal Estuary," *Env Management* 44, 505–523, 2009; JoAnn Burkholder et al., "Impacts to a Coastal River and Estuary from Rupture of a Large Swine Waste Holding Lagoon," *J Env Qual* 26(6) 1451–1466, 1997; JoAnn Burkholder et al., "Impacts of Waste from Concentrated Animal Feeding Operations on Water Quality," *Env Health Perspec* 115(2) 2007.

11. Burkholder et al., "Comprehensive Trend Analysis of Nutrients and Related Variables in a Large Eutrophic Estuary, *Limnol Oceanogr* 51(1), 2006.

12. JoAnn Burkholder, e-mail to author, July 21, 2011.

13. Assateague Coastal Trust, Mar 6, 2012.

14. Kathy Phillips is Assateague Coastkeeper, Maryland. Her title shows she is part of the Waterkeeper Alliance.

15. Kathy Phillips, Assateague Coastkeeper, phone interview with author, August 2011.

16. Hannah Connor, interview conducted in North Carolina in August 2011. Ms. Connor is now a staff attorney for the Humane Society of the United States.

17. JoAnn Burkholder, e-mail to author, July 21, 2011.

18. Maggie Black and Ben Fawcett, *The Last Taboo: Opening the Door on the Global Sanitation Crisis.* London: Earthscan, 2008.

19. "Maximizing Manure's Nutrient Values," *National Hog Farmer*, Feb 10, 2011; Hailin Zhang, *Fertilizer Nutrients in Animal Manure.* OSU, n.d.; *Manure Nutrient Management.* Government of Alberta, 2000.

20. "Common Manure Handling Systems," US EPA, Ag 101, epa.gov, accessed Feb 2012.

21. Don Webb, interview at his home in North Carolina, July 2011.

22. Robbin Marks, *Cesspools of Shame: How Factory Farm Lagoons and Sprayfields Threaten Environmental and Public Health*. Natural Resources Defense Council and the Clean Water Network, 2001.

23. Dennis O'Connor, "Report of the Walkerton Inquiry: The Events of May 2000 and Related Issues," 2002; Murray McQuigge, "The Investigative Report of the Walkerton Outbreak of Waterborne Gastroenteritis," prepared by the Bruce Grey-Owen Sound Health Unit, 2000.

24. McQuigge, 2000, p. iii and 47.

25. O'Connor, 2002, p. 3.

26. Sarah Miller, coordinator and researcher, Canadian Environmental Law Association, phone interview with author, Nov 29, 2011.

27. Extreme weather events have been extensively documented. See IPCC, *Climate Change 2007: The Physical Science Basis, Summary for Policymakers.* p. 8.

28. *Putting Meat on the Table.* Pew Commission, 2008, p. 23.

29. Charles Gerba and James Smith, "Sources of Pathogenic Microorganisms and Their Fate During Land Application of Wastes," *J Env Qual* 34: 42–48, 2005.

30. Pacific Southwest Animal Waste, US Environmental Protection Agency, "What's the Problem?" epa.gov, Mar 6, 2012.

31. Eva Pip, University of Winnipeg, e-mail to author, Dec 2011.

32. Mike Williams, Director, Animal and Poultry Waste Management Center, North Carolina State University, telephone interview, August 2011.

33. Mike Williams, telephone interview August 15, 2011 and e-mail communication, January 2012.

34. "Development of Environmentally Superior Technologies for Swine Waste Management as per Agreements between the Attorney General of North Carolina, Smithfield Foods, Premium Standard Farms, and Frontline Farmers," NC State University, cals.ncsu.edu.

35. Steinfeld et al., *Livestock's Long Shadow* 2006, p. 137.

36. Related to me by Dr. Eva Pip, personal interview in Winnipeg, 2010.

37. Janet Honey, "Manitoba Pig and Pork Industry 2010," Department of Agribusiness and Agricultural Economics, University of Manitoba, Apr 2011.

38. "Environmental Sustainability of Hog Production in Manitoba," Clean Environment Commission (CEC), Dec 2007. Also see reports including "State of Lake Winnipeg 1999–2007," Environment Canada, Manitoba Water Stewardship, Jun 2011.

39. Clean Environment Commission, 2007, p. 85.

40. John Lory, Joe Zulovich, and Charles Fulhage, "Hog Manure and Domestic Wastewater Management Objectives," University of Missouri Extension, 2007, extension.missouri.edu; Kendall Thu, "Industrial Agriculture, Democracy, and the Future," in Ervin, et al., *Beyond Factory Farming: Corporate Hog Barns and the Threat to Public Health, the Environment, and Rural Communities.* Saskatoon: Canadian Centre for Policy Alternatives, 2003.

41. Dr. Pip has authored more than 100 refereed journal articles. Those discussing agricultural threats to Lake Winnipeg include "Littoral Mollusc Communities

and Water Quality in Southern Lake Winnipeg, Manitoba, Canada," *Biodiv and Conserv* 15: 3627–2652, 2006.

42. Eva Pip, "Surface Water Quality in Manitoba with Respect to Six Chemical Parameters, Water Body and Sediment Type and Land Use," *Aquatic Ecosystem Health and Management* 8(2) 195–207, 2005.

43. Eva Pip, "A Review of the Effects of the Livestock Industry on the Environment and Human Health," presentation at Manitoba Livestock 2000 Hearings.

44. From a personal interview with a prairie environmentalist, who expressed the opinion that Dr. Pip "is a heroine and should be given the Rachel Carson award." Rachel Carson was a pioneering scientific researcher who alerted the world to pollution with her groundbreaking book *Silent Spring*. An award in her name is sponsored by the Society of Environmental Toxicology and Chemistry, an environmental research association.

45. "Grassroots Campaign Against Government Moratorium on Pork Industry Gains Momentum," Manitobapork.com, Sept 7, 2011.

46. "Embracing a Sustainable Future," Manitoba Pork Council, Mar 2011.

47. "Beyond Factory Farming," beyondfactoryfarming.org.

48. "Beyond Factory Farming," beyondfactoryfarming.org, accessed Nov 2011.

49. Steinfeld et al., 2006, p. xxii.

50. Harald Menzi et al., "Impacts of Intensive Livestock Production and Manure Management on the Environment," in *Livestock in a Changing Landscape*. Vol I, Steinfeld et al., Island Press, 2010, p. 143.

51. Sierra Club, iowa.sierraclub.org; state.ia.us.

52. Mark Mattson, Lake Ontario Waterkeeper, part of Waterkeepers International, phone interview, August 2011.

53. Jim Miller et al., "Quantity and Quality of Runoff from a Beef Cattle Feedlot in Southern Alberta," *J Env Qual* 33: 1088, 2004.

54. J. Y. M. Johnson et al., "Prevalence of *E. coli* O157:H7 and *Salmonella* spp. in Surface Waters of Southern Alberta and Its Relation to Manure Sources," *Canad J Microbiol* 49: 326–335, 2003.

55. Pollution has been documented by governments, academic researchers, industry, and environmental and animal-welfare groups. Among these, see B.C. government Fact Sheets on minimizing nitrogen and phosphorus pollution from poultry manure at al.gov.bc.ca; Publications by Prof. Hans Schreier at the University of B.C. including "Agricultural Water Policy Challenges in BC," *Policy Options*, Jul–Aug 2009; The industry's Sustainable Poultry Farming Group and its website report, "Evaluation of Options for Fraser Valley Poultry Manure Utilization," 2003; and data from the Vancouver Humane Society at vancouverhumanesociety.bc.ca.

56. Hans Schreier, "Agricultural Water Policy Challenges in B.C.," *Policy Options*, Jul–Aug 2009, p. 50.

57. Schreier, 2009, p. 50. On the issue of excessive nitrates, also see David Schindler, Peter Dillon, and Hans Schreier, "A Review of Anthropogenic Sources of Nitrogen and Their Effects on Canadian Aquatic Systems," *Biogeochemistry* 79: 25–44, 2006.

58. Schreier, 2009.
59. "Aquatic Dead Zones," Earth Observatory, National Aeronautics and Space Administration (NASA), earthobservatory.nasa.gov, Mar 10, 2012.
60. "Livestock Sector Drives Increasing Water Pollution," World Resources Institute, earthtrends.wri.org; "Large 2009 Gulf of Mexico 'Dead Zone' Predicted," sciencedaily.com, 2009.
61. David Molden, ed., *Water for Food, Water for Life: A Comprehensive Assessment of Water Management in Agriculture.* International Water Management Institute (IWMI), Earthscan, 2007; Steinfeld et al., 2006, p. 126.
62. Hans Schreier, interview at his University of B.C. faculty office, October 12, 2011. Also see: D. Molden, ed., *Water for Food.* 2007; M. M. Mekonnen and A. Y. Hoekstra, *The Green, Blue and Grey Water Footprint of Farm Animals and Animal Products.* Vol I: Main Report, Value of Water Research Series no. 48. UNESCO, 2010.
63. Arjen Hoekstra, "The Water Footprint of Animal Products," in D'Silva and Webster, 2010, p. 22–33; A. Y. Hoekstra and A. K. Chapagain, "Water Footprints of Nations: Water Use by People as a Function of Their Consumption Pattern," *Water Resource Management* 21: 35–48, 2007.
64. Steinfeld et al., 2006, p. 126.
65. Lester Brown, *Plan B: 4.0: Mobilizing to Save Civilization.* Earth Policy Institute, NY: Norton, 2009; Also see Fred Pearce, *When the Rivers Run Dry. Water: The Defining Crisis of the 21st Century.* Boston: Beacon Press, 2006.
66. Maude Barlow and Tony Clarke, *Blue Gold: The Battle Against Corporate Theft of the World's Water.* Toronto: M&S, 2002, p. xi.
67. Steinfeld et al., 2006, p. 167.
68. Mekonnen and Hoekstra, 2010, p. 5.
69. Steinfeld et al., p. 129.
70. Ibid., p. 167.
71. Ibid., p. 130.
72. Ibid., p. 127.
73. Ibid., p. 144.
74. Eric Millstone and Tim Lang, *The Atlas of Food: Who Eats What, Where, and Why.* University of California Press, 2008.
75. Steinfeld et al., 2006, p. 179.

Chapter 4

1. There is a large scientific literature on the connection between some of the main illnesses of our time and heavy meat production or consumption. See Barry Popkin, *The World Is Fat.* NY: Avery, 2009; Michael Greger, "The Human/Animal Interface: Emergence and Resurgence of Zoonotic Infectious Diseases," *Critical Reviews in Microbiology* 33: 243–299, 2007; Ellen Silbergeld, Jay Graham, and Lance Price, "Industrial Food Animal Production, Antimicrobial Resistance, and Human Health," *Ann Rev Public Health* 29: 151–169, 2008; Genkinger and Koushik, "Meat Consumption and Cancer Risk," *PLoS Medicine* 4(12) 2007; Campbell and Campbell, *The China Study.* Dallas: Ben-

Bella Books, 2006; Harold Mooney, *Consequences of Livestock Production*. In Steinfeld et al., *Livestock in a Changing Landscape*. Island Press, 2010, p. 67–68; and *Meat Eater's Guide to Climate Change and Health*. Environmental Working Group, 2011.

2. "FDA Finalizes Report on 2006 Spinach Outbreak," FDA news release, Mar 23, 2007. fda.gov.

3. "*E. coli* O157:H7 and other Shiga Toxin-Producing *E. coli* (STEC)," Centers for Disease Control and Prevention. Cdc.gov, accessed Feb 28, 2012. On *E. coli*, *Salmonella* and other deadly bacteria and pathogens in food, see "Factory Farms Are the Reason," Kathy Freston in conversation with Dr. Michael Greger, huffingtonpost.com, Jan 8, 2010, accessed Mar 10, 2012.

4. "*Escherichia coli*: Significance of *E. coli* in Drinking Water," Health Canada. hc-sc.gc.ca, accessed Jun 18, 2010.

5. "FDA Finalizes Report on 2006 Spinach Outbreak," FDA news release, Mar 23, 2007.

6. Sabin Russell, "Spinach *E. coli* Linked to Cattle; Manure on Pasture Had Same Strain As Bacteria in Outbreak," *San Francisco Chronicle*, Oct 13, 2006.

7. Many scientific reports document air quality problems in intensive livestock facilities. See Bassirou Bonfoh et al., "Human Health Hazards Associated with Livestock Production," in Steinfeld et al., *Livestock in a Changing Landscape*. 2010, p. 204 and 206.

8. Bill Paton, "The Smell of Intensive Pig Production on the Canadian Prairies," in Alexander Ervin et al., *Beyond Factory Farming*. CCPA, 2003; *Putting Meat on the Table*. Pew Commission, 2008; Andrew Nikiforuk, "Factory Farming Is Polluting the Water Supply," in James Haley, ed., *Pollution*. Greenhaven Press, 2003; Bonfoh et al., 2010; See also numerous publications from the lab of Dr. Steve Wing, University of North Carolina.

9. *Putting Meat on the Table*. Pew Commission, 2008, p. 17–19; Bonfoh et al., 2010, p. 204.

10. "Iowa Concentrated Animal Feeding Operations Air Quality Study, Final Report," Iowa State University, Feb 2002; Rachel Horton et al., "Malodor as a Trigger of Stress and Negative Mood in Neighbors of Industrial Hog Operations," *Amer J Public Health* 99(S3) 2009; Leah Schinasi et al., "Air Pollution, Lung Function, and the Physical Symptoms in Communities Near Concentrated Swine Feeding Operations," *Epidemiology* 22(2) 2011.

11. Steve Wing and Susanne Wolf, "Intensive Livestock Operations, Health and Quality of Life among Eastern North Carolina Residents," *Env Health Perspec* 108(3) 2000.

12. Bill Paton, "The Smell of Intensive Pig Production on the Canadian Prairies," in Ervin et al., *Beyond Factory Farming*. Saskatoon: CCPA, 2003; Andrew Nikiforuk, "Factory Farming Is Polluting the Water Supply," in James Haley, ed., *Pollution*. Greenhaven Press, 2003; S. Laurent, Parliamentary Research Bureau, Government of Canada, "Rural Canada: Access to Health Care," Dec 2002.

13. Maria Mirabelli et al., "Asthma Symptoms Among Adolescents Who Attend Public Schools That Are Located Near Confined Swine Feeding Operations,"

Pediatrics 118; 66–75, 2006; Julia Barrett, "Hogging the Air: CAFO Emissions Reach into Schools," *Env Health Perspec* 114: A241, Apr 1, 2006.

14. Horton et al., 2009; Paton, 2003; Joel Novek, "Intensive Livestock Operations, Disembedding, and Community Polarization in Manitoba," *Soc Nat Res* 16; 567–581, 2003; M. Tajik et al., "Impact of Odor from Industrial Hog Operations on Daily Living Activities," *New Solutions* 18(2) 2008.

15. Susan Bullers, "Environmental Stressors, Perceived Control, and Health: The Case of Residents Near Large-Scale Hog Farms in E. North Carolina," *Human Ecology* 33(1) 2005.

16. Eva Pip, "A Review of the Effects of the Livestock Industry on the Environment and Human Health," presentation to the Manitoba Livestock 2000 Hearings, Jul 2000, p. 3.

17. Paul Chan, "Outbreak of Avian Influenza A (H5N1) Virus Infection in Hong Kong in 1997," *Clin Infect Dis* 34 (S2) 2002; L. D. Sims et al., "Avian Influenza in Hong Kong 1997–2002," *Avian Dis* 47(3) 2003.

18. Christine Power, "The Source and Means of Spread of the Avian Influenza Virus in the Lower Fraser Valley of B.C. During an Outbreak in the Winter of 2004," Report for CFIA, 2005; Karen Davis, "The Avian Flu Crisis in Canada," United Poultry Concerns, 2005.

19. Steinfeld et al., *Livestock's Long Shadow.* 2006, p. 198.

20. Robert Uhlig, "Ten Million Animals Were Slaughtered in Foot and Mouth Cull," *The Telegraph*, Jan 23, 2002, telegraph.co.uk, accessed Feb 2012.

21. BSE: bovine spongiform encephalopathy; FMD: foot-and-mouth disease; SARS: severe acute respiratory syndrome.

22. Michael Greger, "The Human/Animal Interface: Emergence and Resurgence of Zoonotic Infectious Diseases," *Critical Reviews in Microbiology* 33: 243–299, 2007.

23. 6th International Conference on Emerging Zoonoses, Feb 24–27, 2011. Cancun, Mexico.

24. Babak Pourbohloul et al., "Initial Human Transmission Dynamics of the Pandemic (H1N1) 2009 Virus in North America," *Influenza Resp Viruses* 3(5) 215–222, 2009.

25. Ibid.

26. Ibid.

27. Bryan Walsh, "H1N1 Virus: The First Legal Action Targets a Pig Farm," *Time Magazine*, May 15, 2009.

28. Ibid.

29. World Health Organization, "Pandemic (H1N1) 2009 Update," 108, Jul 9, 2010, who.int.

30. Cathy Holtslander, "Goat Horns Don't Belong on a Pig: Laying the Blame for Swine Flu Where It Belongs," beyondfactoryfarming.org, 2009.

31. Greger, 2007, p. 254; Robert Tauxe "Emerging Food-Borne Pathogens," *Intl J Food Microbio* 78, 31–41, 2002.

32. GRAIN, "A Food System That Kills: Swine Flu Is Meat Industry's Latest Plague," *Against the Grain*, Apr 2009, p. 1, 3.

33. A biological principle holds that genetic diversity helps protect a group of animals or plants against pathology. A diverse group will tend to include members whose genotype(s) decrease(s) their vulnerability to any particular disease agent.
34. These animal welfare issues are extensively documented. See Daniel Imhoff, ed., *The CAFO Reader.* Watershed Media, 2010.
35. James Galloway et al., "International Trade in Meat: The Tip of the Pork Chop," *AMBIO* 36(8) 2007.
36. Greger 2007, p. 252.
37. Ibid., p. 250.
38. Ibid., p. 251.
39. EUROCJD (European Creutzfeldt-Jakob Disease Surveillance Network) eurocjd.ed.ac.uk, accessed Jul 2011.
40. "Mad Cow Disease (BSE) Beyond Factory Farming: Get Informed," beyond factoryfarming.org, 2010; Frédéric Frederic Forge, "Canadian Feed Policy and BSE," Parliamentary Information and Research Service, Govt of Canada, parl.gc.ca, Jul 11, 2005, accessed Feb 2, 2012; Frederic Forge and Jean-Denis Frechette, "Mad Cow Disease and Canada's Cattle Industry," Canadian Parliamentary Information and Research Service, parl.gc.ca, 2005, p. 2.
41. Chad Skelton, "Cattle Feed Contaminated by Animal Parts: Secret Canadian Tests Reveal Proteins in Both Domestic and Imported Feed," *Vancouver Sun,* Dec 16, 2004.
42. European Parliament press release. "Mad Cow Disease: EU Must Maintain Strict Controls, Says Parliament," Jun 7, 2011, europarl.europa.eu.
43. Michael Greger. Interview with health writer Kathy Freston, 2010. Dr. Greger is director of Public Health and Animal Agriculture at the Humane Society of the United States.
44. Greger, 2010.
45. CFIA, "Summary of Feed Drug Clearances," inspection.gc.ca, accessed Mar 3, 2012.
46. FDA, "Animal and Veterinary Green Book Online," fda.gov, accessed Mar 3, 2012.
47. Roxarsone, wolframalpha.com; Canadian Food Inspection Agency, 3-Nitro-4-hydroxyphenylarsonic acid: Roxarsone, inspection.gc.ca; FDA: fda.gov.
48. H. D. Chapman and Z. B. Johnson, "Use of Antibiotics and Roxarsone in Broiler Chickens in the USA: Analysis for the Years 1995 to 2000," *Poultry Science* 81: 356–364, 2002.
49. U.S. Food and Drug Administration Center for Veterinary Medicine. Questions and Answers Regarding 3-Nitro (Roxarsone), fda.gov, 2011.
50. Canada: hc-sc.gc.ca; FDA: fda.gov; Health Canada Veterinary Drugs Directorate, e-mail communication with author, Jan 9, 2012.
51. Tyson Foods said in 2004 that it would stop using Roxarsone.
52. Food and Drug Administration Media Call, Jun 8, 2011. Moderator: Stephanie Yao of FDA. fda.gov; CFIA, inspection.gc.ca.
53. Ibid.

54. For more background and analysis, see David Wallinga, *Playing Chicken: Avoiding Arsenic in Your Meat.* Institute for Agriculture and Trade Policy, 2006.

55. Food and Drug Administration document on PAYLEAN 9 and PAYLEAN 45 (Ractopamine Hydrochloride) Type A Medicated Article for Finishing Swine Apr 25, 2006; CFIA, "Responding to Changing Demands Through Integrated Science" (includes discussion of ractopamine), modified Jun 30, 2011, inspection.gc.ca; Freedom of Information Summary, "Supplemental New Animal Drug Application: Paylean 9 and 45: Ractopamine Hydrochloride. Type a Medicated Article for Finishing Swine," fda.gov, accessed Feb 2012; "Paylean Pays in Canada," payleanpays.ca.

56. Helena Bottemiller, "Dispute Over Drug in Feed Limiting U.S. Meat Exports," Food and Environment Reporting Network, Jan 25, 2012.

57. Canadian Food Inspection Agency (CFIA), "Ractopamine Hydrochloride—MIB #82," inspection.gc.ca," modified Oct 15, 2010, accessed Mar 7, 2012.

58. Ibid.

59. Ibid.

60. That caution appears to have been removed from the website between July and October, 2010, but I have printouts of the earlier version of the site. Canadian Food Inspection Agency (CFIA), "Ractopamine Hydrochloride—MIB #82," inspection.gc.ca," modified Oct 15, 2010.

61. For this wisdom, I pay tribute to the memory of Professor Lewis Seiden, noted scientist, author, and teacher at the University of Chicago.

62. Health Canada, "Questions and Answers—Hormonal Growth Promoters," hc-sc.gc.ca, accessed Mar 10, 2012. The Health Canada site says hormonal growth promoters for beef cattle make the meat leaner, therefore healthier, and also lower beef prices for consumers.

63. Mike Teillet, Manager of Sustainable Development Programs, Manitoba Pork Council, e-mail to author, Dec 6, 2011.

64. centerforfoodsafety.org; inspection.gc.ca.

65. Renee Johnson and Charles Hanrahan, "The U.S.-EU Beef Hormone Controversy," Congressional Research Service, Report for Congress, Dec 6, 2010, crs.gov, p. 1. Also see sustainabletable.org; Janet Raloff, "Hormones: Here's the Beef: Environmental Concerns Re-Emerge Over Steroids Given to Livestock," *Science News* 161(1), Jan 2002.

66. Nicolette Hahn Niman, *Righteous Porkchop: Finding a Life and Good Food Beyond Factory Farms.* 2010, p. 148. Also see "Growth Hormones Fed to Beef Cattle Damage Human Health," Organic Cons Assn., organicconsumers.org, May 2007.

67. "Opposition to the Use of Hormone Growth Promoters in Beef and Dairy Cattle Production," Policy Statement, American Public Health Assn., Nov 10, 2009. "Hormones Used in Livestock Production," Beyond Factory Farming, Petition no. 203 to Canadian government, oag-bvg.gc.ca, May 2007; Opinion of the Scientific Committee on Veterinary Measures relating to Public Health: "Assessment of Potential Risks to Human Health from Hormone Residues in Bovine Meat and Meat Products, European Commission," Apr 30, 1999, p. 72.

68. "Opposition to the Use of Hormone Growth Promoters in Beef and Dairy Cattle Production," policy statement, American Public Health Assn., Nov 10, 2009, apha.org.
69. "Hormones Used in Livestock Production," Beyond Factory Farming, petition, 2007.
70. In this case, the government's scientific reference was a study funded partly by Ontario Pork: A. Lorenzen et al., "Persistence and Pathways of Testosterone Dissipation in Agricultural Soil," *J Env Qual* 34: 854–860, 2004. Meanwhile, other studies are sometimes funded by organizations with alternative points of view. For background from a citizen group, see "Hormones Used in Livestock Production," beyondfactoryfarming.org, 2007.
71. "Assessment of Potential Risks to Human Health from Hormone Residues in Bovine Meat and Meat Products," European Commission, Apr 30, 1999, p. 72.
72. "WTO Panel Cases to Which Canada Is a Party," international.gc.ca, accessed Mar 7, 2012. Also see sustainabletable.org on hormones.
73. Dennis Bueckert, "Beef Hormones Linked to Premature Onset of Puberty and Breast Cancer," Canadian Press, organicconsumers.org, 1999.
74. Zosia Bielski, "Obesity Linked to More Girls Hitting Puberty As Young As 7, Study Shows," *Globe and Mail*, Aug 9, 2010.
75. Frank Biro et al., "Pubertal Assessment Method and Baseline Characteristics in a Mixed Longitudinal Study of Girls," *Pediatrics*. Published online Aug 9, 2010, pediatricsdigest.mobi.
76. Joel Fuhrman, MD, "Girls' Early Puberty: What Causes It, and How to Avoid It," *The Huffington Post*, May 6, 2011.
77. CFIA: Steroidal Growth Promotants (licensed for use in calves, heifers and steers), inspection.gc.ca; FDA, "Steroid Hormone Implants Used for Growth in Food-Producing Animals," fda.gov.
78. Anke Gunther et al., "Dietary Protein Intake Throughout Childhood Is Associated with the Timing of Puberty," *J Nutrition* 140: 565–571, 2010. Also see studies cited in Imogen Rogers et al., 2010, p. 2059.
79. Imogen Rogers et al., "Diet Throughout Childhood and Age at Menarche in a Contemporary Cohort of British Girls," *Public Health Nutrition* 13(12) 2052–2063, 2010, p. 2057.
80. Dr. Imogen Rogers, University of Brighton, UK, e-mail to author, February 6, 2012.
81. Sandra Cesario and Lisa Hughes, "Precocious Puberty: A Comprehensive Review of Literature," *AWHONN* 36(3) 2007.
82. Eili Klein, David Smith, and Ramanan Laxminarayan, "Hospitalizations and Deaths Caused by MRSA, U.S., 1999–2005," *Emerging Infectious Diseases* 13 (12), Dec 2007; Centers for Disease Control: cdc.gov; Salynn Boyles, "More U.S. Deaths from MRSA Than AIDS," WebMD Health, Oct 16, 2007.
83. "MRSA Statistics," Centers for Disease Control, Apr 8, 2011, cdc.gov, accessed Mar 7, 2012.
84. Ralph Loglisci, "New FDA Numbers Reveal Food Animals Consume Lion's Share of Antibiotics," Center for a Livable Future, Dec 23, 2010, livablefuture

blog.com; Andrew Gunther, "The FDA Fails the Public on Antibiotics Once Again," *The Huffington Post*, Jan 9, 2012; David Kirby, "MRSA in Meat: Why No Recall?" huffingtonpost.com, Sep 15, 2010.

85. "Antibiotics Use in Hogs," Corporate Responsibility Summary Report, 2010/11, Smithfield Foods, p. 27.

86. World Health Organization, "Information for Farmers, Veterinarians and Veterinary or Food Safety Authorities (on Antibiotics)," euro.who.int, Apr 7, 2011, accessed Feb 2012.

87. FDA, "The Judicious Use of Medically Important Drugs in Food-Producing Animals," Food and Drug Administration Center for Veterinary Medicine, Jun 28, 2010.

88. Tara Smith et al., "MRSA Strain ST398 Is Present in Midwestern U.S. Swine and Swine Workers," *PLoS ONE* 4(1) e4258, 2009.

89. Ashley O'Brien et al., "MRSA in Conventional and Alternative Retail Pork Products," *PLoS ONE* 7(1), plosone.org, Jan, 2012.

90. Ellen Silbergeld, J. Graham, and L. Price, "Industrial Food Production, Antimicrobial Resistance, and Human Health," *Ann Rev Public Health* 29: 151–169, 2008.

91. jhsph.edu/faculty/directory/profile/3806/Silbergeld/Ellen. Mar 7, 2012.

92. Silbergeld et al., 2008, p. 153.

93. Aqeel Ahmad et al., "Insects in Confined Swine Operations Carry a Large Antibiotic-Resistant and Potentially Virulent Enterococcal Community," BMC Microbiology, published online Jan 26, 2011, biomedcentral.com.

94. Lucie Dutil et al., "Ceftiofur Resistance in *Salmonella enterica* Serovar Heidelberg from Chicken Meat and Humans, Canada," *Emerging Infectious Diseases* 16 (1) Jan 2010; "Salmonella Heidelberg: Ceftiofur-Related Resistance in Human and Retail Chicken Isolates," Public Health Agency of Canada, 2007 and update, 2009.

95. Silbergeld, 2008, p. 158.

96. Silbergeld, 2008, p. 154–157.

97. Ali Khan, Assistant Surgeon General, Centers for Disease Control and Prevention, testimony before subcommittee on health, U.S. House of Representatives, Jul 14, 2010.

98. Randy Shore, "B.C. Poultry Industry Warned to Halt Use of Antibiotic," *Vancouver Sun*, Nov 25, 2011, p. 1.

99. Centers for Disease Control, "Achievements in Public Health, 1900–1999," cdc.gov; Marion Nestle, *Food Politics*. University of California Press, 2002, p. 2–3.

100. Centers for Disease Control, cdc.gov/nchs.

101. "The Top Ten Causes of Death," World Health Organization Fact Sheet no. 310, updated Jun 2011, who.int.

102. Amy Anderson et al., "Dietary Patterns and Survival of Older Adults," *J Amer Dietetic Assn* 111(1), Jan 2011.

103. Marion Nestle, *What to Eat*. 2006, p. 146; "Nutrition and Healthy Eating: Meatless Meals: The Benefits of Eating Less Meat," Mayo Clinic, Sept 16, 2011,

mayoclinic.com, accessed Mar 7, 2012; Gary Fraser, "Vegetarian Diets: What Do We Know of Their Effects on Common Chronic Diseases?" *Am J Clin Nutr*, Mar 25, 2009.

104. Michael Pollan, *In Defense of Food: An Eater's Manifesto.* NY: Penguin, 2008, p. 182. Mr. Pollan's observations about overeating help inform his credo for health: "Eat food, not too much, mostly plants."

105. McMichael et al., 2007, p. 5.

106. World Health Organization, "Obesity and Overweight," Fact Sheet no. 311, who.int, Mar 2011.

107. David Pimentel and Marcia Pimentel, "Sustainability of Meat-Based and Plant-Based Diets and the Environment," *Am J Clin Nutr* 78: 660S–663S, 2003, p. 661S.

108. Barry Popkin, *The World Is Fat.* 2009; Derek Yach et al., "The Global Burden of Chronic Disease," *JAMA* 291(21) 2004.

109. "Obesity and Overweight: Data for the U.S. (2010)," Centers for Disease Control and Prevention, Atlanta, Georgia.

110. "Obesity Update 2012," Organization for Economic Cooperation and Development (OECD), Feb 21, 2012, oecd.org.

111. Margaret Shields et al., "Adult Obesity Prevalence in Canada and the U.S.," data brief from the National Center for Health Statistics, Centers for Disease Control, cdc.gov/nchs, accessed Mar 7, 2011.

112. T. Colin Campbell and Thomas M. Campbell II, *The China Study.* BenBella Books, 2006.

113. Marion Nestle, *Food Politics: How the Food Industry Influences Nutrition and Health.* Berkeley: University of California Press, 2002, p 3.

114. Caroline Mayer, "U.S. Snack-Food Makers on a Fitness Kick," Thestandard.com.hk, Nov 26, 2005.

115. McMichael et al., 2007; Popkin, 2009.

116. Mark Bittman, *Food Matters: A Guide to Conscious Eating.* Simon & Schuster, 2009; Mark Bittman, "Bad Food? Tax It, and Subsidize Vegetables," *New York Times*, p. R1, Jul 23, 2011.

117. Marion Nestle, *What to Eat.* 2006; Polly Walker et al., "Public Health Implications of Meat Production and Consumption," *Public Health Nutrition* 8(4) 348–356, 2005; Campbell and Campbell, *The China Study.* 2006.

118. Polly Walker et al., 2005, p. 348.

119. Centers for Disease Control. cdc.gov; Also CDC-INFO e-mail August 10, 2011.

120. Heart and Stroke Foundation, heartandstroke.com, accessed Feb 2012.

121. Marion Nestle, *What to Eat.* 2006; Vesanto Melina and Brenda Davis, *Becoming Vegetarian.* Wiley, 2003.

122. Sharon Friel et al., "Public Health Benefits of Strategies to Reduce Greenhouse Gas Emissions: Food and Agriculture," *The Lancet* 374(9706) 2016-2025, Dec 12, 2009.

123. Heart and Stroke Foundation, "Stroke Prevention, 2011," heartandstroke.com.

124. *Food, Nutrition, Physical Activity, and the Prevention of Cancer: A Global Perspective.* World Cancer Research Fund and American Institute for Cancer

Research, 2007; International Agency for Research on Cancer, World Health Organization, 2005.

125. Amanda Cross et al., "A Prospective Study of Red and Processed Meat Intake in Relation to Cancer Risk," *PLoS Med* 4(12) Dec 2007.

126. Physicians Committee for Responsible Medicine, "The Cancer Project," cancer project.org.

127. Susanna Larsson, Nicola Orsini, and Alicja Wolk, "Processed Meat Consumption and Stomach Cancer Risk: A Meta-Analysis," *J Natl Cancer Inst* 98 (15) 1078–1087, 2006, p. 1085. For further studies about processed meats, see the meta-analysis by epidemiologists at Sweden's Karolinska Institute, showing a link between eating processed meats and getting stomach cancer. Meanwhile, the U.S. National Cancer Institute has demonstrated that red and processed meats can increase risk of disease in other organs.

128. E. F. Taylor et al., "Meat Consumption and Risk of Breast Cancer in the UK Women's Cohort Study," *Brit J Cancer* 96: 1139–1146, 2007.

129. "Food, Nutrition, Physical Activity, and the Prevention of Cancer: A Global Perspective," World Cancer Research Fund and American Institute for Cancer Research, 2007. dietandcancerreport.org, accessed Feb 10, 2012.

130. "Food, Nutrition, Physical Activity, and the Prevention of Cancer: A Global Perspective," Second Expert Report, recommendations, World Cancer Research Fund and the American Institute for Cancer Research, dietandcancer report.org, Mar 10, 2012.

131. Steinfeld et al., 2006, p. 158.

132. Ibid.

133. "National Diabetes Information Clearing House," National Institutes of Health, 2011; "National Diabetes Fact Sheet," Centers for Disease Control, 2011, cdc.gov.

134. "National Diabetes Fact Sheet," Centers for Disease Control, 2011.

135. Yiqing Song et al., "A Prospective Study of Red Meat Consumption and Type 2 Diabetes in Middle-Aged and Elderly Women: The Women's Health Study," diabetesjournals.org, 2004; Rob Van Dam et al., "Dietary Fat and Meat Intake in Relation to Risk of Type 2 Diabetes in Men," *Diabetes Care* 25 (3) 417–424, 2002.

136. "The Lady's Brunch Burger," Paula Deen, 2008, foodnetwork.com.

137. diabetesinanewlight.com, nytimes.com, Mar 7, 2012.

138. T. Colin Campbell and Thomas Campbell II, *The China Study*. BenBella Books, 2006.

139. Campbell and Campbell, *The China Study*. 2006.

140. Campbell and Campbell, *The China Study*. 2006, p. 233, p. 69–108.

141. BC Cancer Agency, bccancer.bc.ca, revised Nov 16, 2005, accessed Mar 7, 2012.

142. *Food, Nutrition, Physical Activity, and the Prevention of Cancer: A Global Perspective.* World Cancer Research Fund and American Institute for Cancer Research, 2007, p. iv and xix.

143. Personal interview with Rancher Francis Gardner, his wife Bonnie and

daughter Sarah, and neighbor Gordon Cartwright, at Mount Sentinel Ranch in southern Alberta, August 10, 2010.

Chapter 5

1. Elsie Herring, personal interview conducted in North Carolina, August 14, 2011.
2. Steve Wing et al., "Environmental Injustice in North Carolina's Hog Industry," *Env Health Perspec* 108(3) 2000; also see Jennifer Norton et al., "Race, Wealth and Solid Waste Facilities in North Carolina," *Env Health Perspec* 115(9) 2007, showing that waste facilities are disproportionately located in communities of color and low wealth.
3. Naeema Muhammed, community organizer, North Carolina Environmental Justice Network. Personal interview in North Carolina, July 13, 2011.
4. "Hogs' Halt," *The Economist*, Sept 18, 1997; "Lawmaker Says Voters Want More Regulations for Hog Farms."*Wilmington Morning Star*, Apr 14, 1997.
5. Kendall Thu, "Industrial Agriculture, Democracy, and the Future," in *Beyond Factory Farming*. Ervin et al., CCPA, 2003, p. 10.
6. Steve Wing and Susanna Wolf, "Intensive Livestock Operations, Health and Quality of Life Among Eastern North Carolina Residents," *Env Health Perspec* 2000, p. 233; Rachel Horton et al., "Malodor as a Trigger of Stress and Negative Mood in Neighbors of Industrial Hog Operations," *Am J Public Health* 99(S3), 2009.
7. William Weida, "The ILO and Depopulation of Rural Agricultural Areas: Implications for Rural Economies in Canada and the U.S.," National Conference on Intensive Livestock Operations, Saskatoon, Saskatchewan, Nov 8, 2002. Dr. Weida published an essay under the same title in Ervin et al., eds., *Beyond Factory Farming*. 2003; John Kilpatrick, "Concentrated Animal Feeding Operations and Proximate Property Values," *The Appraisal Journal* LXIX (3) Jul 2001.
8. William Weida, "The ILO and Depopulation of Rural Agricultural Areas," in Ervin et al., *Beyond Factory Farming*, p. 111–140.
9. Joel Novek, "Intensive Livestock Operations, Disembedding, and Community Polarization in Manitoba," *Soc Nat Res* 16: 567–581, 2003.
10. Novek, 2003, p. 576.
11. Novek, 2003; Ervin et al., *Beyond Factory Farming*, 2003; *Putting Meat on the Table*. Pew Commission, 2008, p. 43.
12. Patrick McCormally, "Right-to-Farm Legislation in Canada: Environment Probe," probeinternational.org, Jul 2007; State Environmental Resource Center, "Issue: CAFO Zoning," serconline.org, Mar 7, 2012.
13. Thomas Pawlick, *The War in the Country*. Vancouver: Greystone, 2009, p. 1.
14. Mark Bittman, *Food Matters: A Guide to Conscious Eating*. NY: Simon & Schuster, 2009, p. 21.
15. Statistics Canada 2008, quoted in *Regina Leader-Post*, Dec 3, 2008, "Number of Farmers Continues Steep Decline," canada.com.

16. National Farmers' Union 2010b, "Free Trade: Is It Working for Farmers? Comparing 1988 to 2010," *Union Farmer Monthly* 60(2) Jun 2010.

17. Kendall Thu, "Industrial Agriculture, Democracy, and the Future," in *Beyond Factory Farming*, Ervin et al., 2003, p. 9–28.

18. *Dairy Facts 2010.* International Dairy Foods Assn., Washington, DC, 2010, p. 17.

19. *Factory Farm Nation: How America Turned Its Livestock Farms into Factories.* Food and Water Watch, 2010, p. 4.

20. *Factory Farm Nation*, 2010.

21. For the 100-year comparison, see Eric Schlosser's foreword to the 2006 Penguin re-issue of the 1906 book by Upton Sinclair, *The Jungle*. p. xii. Also see John Anderson and Darren Hudson, "Acquisitions and Integration in the Beef Industry," Agricultural and Applied Economics Assn., 2008.

22. "Anti-Trust Law, Corporate Concentration and the Meat Processing Industry," Reforming Industrial Animal Agriculture, Pew Charitable Trusts, Fact Sheet, Jan 28, 2011; Mary Hendrickson and William Heffernan, *Concentration of Agricultural Markets*. Dept of Rural Sociology, University of Missouri, 2007.

23. David Kirby, *Animal Factory*. St. Martin's Press, 2010, p. xiv.

24. Food policy expert Rod MacRae, professor of Environmental Studies at York University in Toronto, has written that Canada's food system is highly oligopolistic. See Rod MacRae, "A Joined-Up Food Policy for Canada," *J Hunger and Environ Nutrition* 6(4) 424–457, 2011; Rod MacRae, "Policy Failure in the Canadian Food System, International Development Research Centre, Ottawa," web.idrc.ca, 1999.

25. U.S. Dept of Justice brief on an anti-trust action against Smithfield Foods, 2003.

26. Murphy-Brown, "Contract Growers," murphybrownllc.com, accessed Feb 2012; "Anti-Trust Law, Corporation Concentration, and the Meat Processing Industry," Pew Environmental Group, pewenvironment.org, Jan 2011.

27. David Moeller, *Livestock Production Contracts: Risks for Family Farmers.* Farmers' Legal Action Group, St. Paul, Minn. 2003.

28. Steve Martinez and Kelly Zering, "Pork Quality and the Role of Market Organization," USDA Economic Research Service, Oct 2004.

29. UN FAO, "Save and Grow," fao.org, 2011; "Small Farms Key to Global Food Security, UN Says," Reuters Africa, Jul 5, 2011; Interview with Peter Rosset of Food First, The Institute for Food and Development Policy, "The Case for Small Farms," *Multinational Monitor* 21(7), 2000, multinationalmonitor.org, accessed Mar 3, 2012; Peter Hazell, *Five Big Questions about Five Hundred Million Small Farms*. Conference on New Directions for Smallholder Agriculture, International Fund for Agricultural Development, Rome, Jan 2011.

30. Brian Halweil, *Eat Here: Reclaiming Homegrown Pleasures in a Global Supermarket*. NY: Norton, 2004, p. 75.

31. Peter Rosset, *The Multiple Functions and Benefits of Small Farm Agriculture.* Food First Policy Brief no. 4, Sept 1999, p. 1.

32. Peter Rosset interview, *Multinational Monitor* 2000.

33. Miguel Altieri, "Agroecology, Small Farms, and Food Sovereignty," *Monthly Review* 61(3) Jul/Aug, 2009.
34. World Economic and Social Survey 2011, *The Great Green Technological Transformation*. United Nations Dept of Economic and Social Affairs, NY, 2011.
35. "Save and Grow," UN FAO, fao.org, May 2011.
36. Colleen and her husband, John Weatherhead, operate Waratah Downs Organic Farm near Ottawa, in southern Ontario.
37. *Losing Our Grip: How a Corporate Farmland Buy-Up, Rising Farm Debt, and Agribusiness Financing of Inputs Threaten Family Farms and Food Sovereignty.* National Farmers' Union of Canada, 2010.
38. John Ikerd, "Corporate Livestock Production: Implications for Rural North America," in *Beyond Factory Farming*, Ervin et al., CCPA, 2003, p. 30.
39. Ibid., p. 33.
40. Ibid.
41. *Beyond Factory Farming.* 2003, p. 3; Fred Tait, "Pork, Politics and Power," in *Beyond Factory Farming*, p. 53.
42. *Beyond Factory Farming*, p. 3.
43. Eric Schlosser, *Fast Food Nation.* Perennial, 2002.
44. Thu, in *Beyond Factory Farming*, p. 15.
45. *What's on Your Plate? The Hidden Costs of Industrial Animal Agriculture in Canada.* Toronto: World Society for the Protection of Animals, 2012; *Putting Meat on the Table.* Pew Commission, 2008.
46. *A Place in the Choir.* Folk song written in 1977 by American musician Bill Staines. Originally "All God's Critters Got a Place in the Choir," it was recorded as "All God's creatures..."
47. Donald Bixby, "Old MacDonald Had Biodiversity," in *The CAFO Reader*. Daniel Imhoff, ed., Watershed Media, 2010.
48. Daniel Imhoff, "Consequences of Diversity Loss," in *The CAFO Reader*. 2010, p. 191.
49. *The CAFO Reader*. p. 193.
50. "Global Plan of Action for Animal Genetic Resources and the Interlaken Declaration," FAO, 2007.
51. Michael Pollan, *The Botany of Desire.* Random House, 2001.
52. Dan Koeppel, *Banana: The Fate of the Fruit That Changed the World.* Plume, 2009.
53. Dan Koeppel, "Can This Fruit Be Saved?" *Popular Science*, Aug 2005.
54. Claire Thompson, "Something to Be Thankful for: Real Turkeys Make a Comeback," *Grist*, Nov 14, 2011, grist.org, accessed Mar 7, 2012.
55. Good Shepherd Poultry, goodshepherdpoultryranch.com.
56. Don Webb, personal interview at his home in North Carolina, August 15, 2011.
57. Jonathan Safran Foer, *Eating Animals.* Little, Brown, 2009.
58. Robert Zimdahl, *Agriculture's Ethical Horizon.* Elsevier, 2012.
59. Peter Singer, "Animal Liberation: Vegetarianism as Protest," in Steve Sapontzis, *Food for Thought: The Debate Over Eating Meat.* Prometheus, 2004.

60. Eleanor Boyle, "Neuroscience and Animal Sentience," Compassion in World Farming, ciwf.org.uk, 2009.

61. Thanks to Jonathan Balcombe for his documentation of animals' capacity for pleasure, e.g., in *The Exultant Ark: A Pictorial Tour of Animal Pleasure*. University of California Press, 2012.

62. Vancouver Humane Society, Eat Less Meat campaign, vancouverhumane society.bc.ca, Mar 4, 2012.

63. James McWilliams, speech at the National Conference to End Factory Farming, Arlington, VA, Oct 2011. Mr. McWilliams is author of *Just Food: Where Locavores Get It Wrong and How We Can Truly Eat Responsibly*. Little, Brown, 2009.

64. This position is argued by meat company representatives and supporters of intensive livestock systems. Indeed, there is evidence that animals raised intensively indoors have reduced incidence of some parasites. See: Peter Davies, "Intensive Swine Production and Pork Safety," *Foodborne Pathogens and Disease* 8(2) 189–201, 2011.

65. Joyce Holmes of Empire Valley Ranch, B.C., e-mail to author, November, 2011.

Chapter 6

1. The In Vitro Meat Consortium, invitromeat.org, accessed Mar 3, 2012; Also see *World Livestock 2011*. UN FAO, 2011, p. 81; and Michael Specter, "Test-Tube Burgers," *The New Yorker*, May 23, 2011.

2. *World Livestock 2011*. UN FAO, 2011, p. 81.

3. Henning Steinfeld and Pierre Gerber, "Livestock Production and the Global Environment: Consume Less or Produce Better?" *PNAS* 107(43) 2010, p. 18238.

4. Tim Lang, David Barling, and Martin Caraher, *Food Policy: Integrating Health, Environment and Society*. Oxford University Press, 2009.

5. Boris Johnson, "Save the Planet by Cutting Down on Meat? That's Just a Load of Bull," *The Telegraph*, Sept 9, 2008.

6. College of Agricultural Sciences, Penn State, "Meat Heaven and Dirty Jobs: Making 5th Annual Meat-In Day a Success," das.psu.edu, Mar 16, 2011, accessed Dec, 2011.

7. Mike Archer, "Ordering the Vegetarian Meal? There's More Animal Blood on Your Hands," *The Conversation*, theconversation.edu.au, Dec 2011, accessed Jan 2012.

8. Joyce Holmes, Empire Valley Beef, detailed e-mail to the author, November 2011.

9. McMichael and Butler, 2010; Walker et al., 2005; Wirsenius and Hedenus, 2010; *World Livestock 2011*. UN FAO, 2011.

10. Steinfeld et al., *Livestock's Long Shadow*, 2006; Garnett, 2010; Reganold et al., 2011; Steinfeld et al., *Livestock in a Changing Landscape*, 2010; MacMillan and Durrant, 2009.

11. Steinfeld and Gerber, 2010.

12. For example, the intergovernmental European Cooperation in Science and

Technology held a meeting of top policy experts on March 16, 2012, in Amsterdam, entitled "Exploratory Workshop: Sustainable Protein Supply."

13. B. P. Weidema et al., "Environmental Improvement Potentials of Meat and Dairy Products," European Commission Joint Research Centre, 2008, p.7.

14. Steinfeld et al., 2006.

15. MacMillan and Durrant, *Livestock Consumption and Climate Change: A Framework for Dialogue*. Food Ethics Council and World Wildlife Fund, Sep 2009; McMichael et al., 2007; Audsley et al., 2009; Tara Garnett, "Livestock-Related Greenhouse Gas Emissions: Impacts and Options for Policy Makers," *Env Sci Pol* 12: 491–503, 2009.

16. Nathan Pelletier and Peter Tyedmers, "Forecasting Potential Global Environmental Costs of Livestock Production," *PNAS* 107(43) 18371–18374, Oct 26, 2010. Dalhousie University is located in Halifax, Nova Scotia.

17. Kari Hamerschlag, *Meat Eater's Guide to Climate Change and Health*. Environmental Working Group, Jul 2011, ewg.org.

18. MacMillan and Durrant, 2009, p. 10.

19. Al Gore, youtube.com, Mar 3, 2012.

20. Barry Popkin, "Reducing Meat Consumption Has Multiple Benefits for the World's Health," *Arch Intern Med* 169(6) 543–545, 2009.

21. D'Silva and Webster, eds., *The Meat Crisis*. 2010; Lang, Barling, and Caraher, *Food Policy*. 2009.

22. Daniel Imhoff, *Food Fight: The Citizens' Guide to the Next Food and Farm Bill*. Watershed Media, 2012.

23. Lang, Barling, and Caraher, 2009; MacRae, 2011; Peter Ladner, *The Urban Food Revolution: Changing the Way We Feed Cities*. Gabriola Island, B.C.: New Society Publishers, 2011.

24. meatlessmonday.com, Mar 3, 2012.

25. Meatless Monday project associate Tami O'Neill, e-mail to author February, 2012.

26. meatlessmonday.com.

27. meatlessmonday.com; epicurious.com, Mar 3, 2012.

28. *Climate Protection Action Plan*. City of Cincinnati, Jun 19, 2008, p. 209.

29. Swedish National Food Agency, *The National Food Administration's Environmentally Effective Food Choices*. May 15, 2009, Proposal notified to the EU.

30. Monika Pearson, Nutritionist, Food Data Division, Swedish National Food Administration, e-mail to author, February 10, 2012.

31. "Sweden and Environmentally Friendly Dietary Guidelines: Life, Law, Politics and the Environment," czarnezki.com, Sept 9, 2011.

32. Swedish National Food Agency, *The National Food Administration's Environmentally Effective Food Choices*. 2009, p.1.

33. Swedish National Food Agency, se/en-gb, Mar 7, 2012.

34. Friends of the Earth, "Healthy Planet Eating," 2010, p. 1.

35. Public Health Assn. of Australia, *A Future for Food: Healthy. Sustainable. Fair.* Feb 20, 2012.

36. Thanks to food writer Michael Pollan for popularizing the term "omnivore" to describe the human condition of being able to survive on plant, or meat, or mixed diets.
37. Allan Nation, foreword to Joel Salatin's, *Folks, This Ain't Normal*, 2011, p. ix.
38. Matthew Scully, "Fear Factories: The Case for Compassionate Conservatism—for Animals," in *The CAFO Reader*. 2010, p. 15.
39. Mike Williams, "Development of Environmentally Superior Technologies: Phase 3 Report for Technology Determinations per Agreements Between the Attorney General of North Carolina and Smithfield Foods, Premium Standard Farms, and Frontline Farmers," Animal and Poultry Waste Management Center, NC State University, cals.ncsu.edu, Mar 8, 2006.
40. The project was partly funded by multinational pork producer Smithfield Foods.
41. Doug Gurian-Sherman, *Raising the Steaks: Global Warming and Pasture-Raised Beef Production in the U.S.* Union of Concerned Scientists, 2011.
42. Smith et al., 2008; MacMillan and Durrant, *Livestock Consumption*, 2009.
43. Dennis Treacy, executive vice-president corporate affairs and chief sustainability officer, Smithfield Foods, telephone interview with the author, February 8, 2012.
44. smithfieldcommitments.com, Mar 3, 2012.
45. Pete Smith et al., "Greenhouse Gas Mitigation in Agriculture," *Phil Trans R Soc B* 363: 789–813, 2008, p. 807.
46. J. P. Reganold et al., "Transforming U.S. Agriculture," *Science* 332: 670–671, May 6, 2011.
47. Human slavery was abolished in the United States with the passage of the 13th amendment to the Constitution in 1865.
48. Mark Bittman, "We're Eating Less Meat. Why?" Opinionator, *New York Times*, Jan 10, 2012.
49. Erik De Bakker and Hans Dagevos, "Reducing Meat Consumption in Today's Consumer Society: Questioning the Citizen-Consumer Gap," *J Agric Enviro Ethics*, Sept 2011.
50. Epicurious, "Back to the Future: Ten Food Trends to Watch over the Next Decade," epicurious.com, 2010.
51. Sustain, sustainweb.org, 2011.
52. Weber and Matthews, 2008, p. 3508.
53. Rosamond Naylor et al., "Losing the Links Between Livestock and Land," *Science* 310, Dec 9, 2005.
54. McMichael et al., 2007.
55. Dr. Anthony McMichael, e-mail to author, November, 2011.
56. David Pimentel and Marcia Pimentel, "Sustainability of Meat-Based and Plant-Based Diets and the Environment," *Am J Clin Nutr* 78: 660S-3S, 2003; David Pimentel et al., "Reducing Energy Inputs in the United States Food System," *Human Ecology* 36(4) 459–471, 2008.
57. Pimentel et al., 2008; Pimentel and Pimentel, 2003.
58. Amanda Cross et al., "A Prospective Study of Red and Processed Meat Intake

in Relation to Cancer Risk," *PLoS Medicine* 4(12) Dec 2007; HealthDay, Dec 11, 2007.

59. Dr. Amanda Cross, personal communication, e-mail to author, Jan 2012. Also see Cross et al., 2007; Also see other studies by Dr. Cross and colleagues, e.g., Cross et al., "Meat Consumption and Risk of Esophageal and Gastric Cancer in a Large Prospective Study," *Am J Gastroenterol* 106(3) 432–42, 2011.

60. World Cancer Research Fund and American Institute for Cancer Research, *Food, Nutrition, Physical Activity, and the Prevention of Cancer: A Global Perspective.* n.d. dietandcancerreport.org, accessed Feb 2012.

61. "Healthy Planet Eating," 2010.

62. Friends of the Earth (FOE) and Compassion in World Farming, "Eating the Planet? How We Can Feed the World Without Trashing It." Nov 2009; FOE, "Healthy Planet Eating: How Lower Meat Diets Can Save Lives and the Planet," 2010.

63. Compassion in World Farming, "Global Warming: Climate Change and Farm Animal Welfare," ciwf.org, 2007, p. 5.

64. Jonathon Porritt, in *The Meat Crisis.* 2010, p. 278.

65. Graham Hill, "Weekday Vegetarian," ted.com/talks/graham_hill, Mar 8, 2012.

66. For a discussion of effective community-based social marketing, see Doug McKenzie-Mohr, *Fostering Sustainable Behavior*, 3rd ed. Gabriola Island, B.C.: New Society Publishers, 2011.

67. Vaclav Smil, "Worldwide Transformation of Diets, Burdens of Meat Production and Opportunities for Novel Food Proteins," *Enz and Microb Tech* 30: 305–311, 2002, p. 310. Dr. Smil's new book will be *Eating Meat: Evolution and Consequences of Human Carnivory.* See more of his works at vaclavsmil.com.

Chapter 7

1. Annie Somerville, Executive Chef, Greens Restaurant, San Francisco. Telephone interview, August 17, 2011.

2. In the context of the meat problem, authors Erik De Bakker and Hans Dagevos discuss the necessity for consumers to be agents of change in "Reducing Meat Consumption in Today's Consumer Society: Questioning the Citizen-Consumer Gap," *J Agric Enviro Ethics* 2011.

3. "The State of Food and Agriculture: Livestock in the Balance," UN FAO, 2009, p. 10.

4. Finlo Rohrer, "China Drinks Its Milk," BBC News, Aug 7, 2007, news.bbc.co.uk.

5. Steinfeld et al., 2006.

6. Steinfeld et al., 2006; McMichael and Butler, 2010.

7. "The State of Food and Agriculture: Livestock in the Balance," UN FAO, 2009; Steinfeld et al., 2006.

8. China Sustainable Agriculture Innovation Network, sainonline.org.

9. Basia Romanowicz, World Society for the Protection of Animals. Telephone interview with author, September 2011.

10. Article on Vandana Shiva and her work in India on sustainable agriculture, vandanashiva.org.
11. *Meat Eater's Guide.* 2011.
12. Jonathan Foley et al., "Solutions for a Cultivated Planet," *Nature* 2011.
13. Examples include The Black Hoof (theblackhoof.com) in Toronto, and Incanto (incanto.biz) in San Francisco.
14. For some ideas, see Lyall Watson's *The Whole Hog: Exploring the Extraordinary Potential of Pigs.* Profile, 2004; and Fergus Henderson's *Nose to Tail Eating: A Kind of British Cooking.* Bloomsbury, 2004.
15. Marion Nestle, *What to Eat.* 2006, p. 165.
16. Canadian Food Inspection Agency (CFIA), "Composition, Quality, Quantity and Origin Claims," inspection.gc.ca. Updated Jan 5, 2012, accessed Mar 11, 2012.
17. Union of Concerned Scientists, fact sheet, ucsusa.org, 2009, accessed Jan 2012.
18. Organic Trade Association, ota.com.
19. Local Food Plus, localfoodplus.ca, accessed Feb 2012.
20. Certified Humane, "Humane Farm Animal Care," certifiedhumane.org, accessed Mar 6, 2012.
21. "American Welfare Approved," animalwelfareapproved.org, accessed Mar 6, 2012.
22. Lester Brown, founder of the Washington-based Worldwatch Institute, "The New Geopolitics of Food," *Foreign Policy*, May/Jun 2011.
23. Michael Pollan, *In Defense of Food.* Penguin, 2008 p. 187–188; and "Big Food vs Big Insurance," Op-Ed, *New York Times* 2009.
24. Global Animal Partnership, "The 5-Step Program," outlines their 5-Step Animal Welfare Rating Standards, globalanimalpartnership.org, accessed Mar 8, 2012.
25. John Mackey, CEO, Whole Foods, "Taxpayers," in *Gristle: From Factory Farms to Food Safety.* Moby and Miyun Park, eds., NY: The New Press, 2010, p. 25.
26. Harris/Decima conducted two surveys for the Vancouver Humane Society, in 2009 and 2010, both of which showed that about 72% of Canadians would pay more for farm animal products if such foods were certified as humane.
27. Ekin Birol, Devesh Roy, and Maximo Torero, "How Safe Is My Food? Assessing the Effect of Information and Credible Certification on Consumer Demand for Food Safety in Developing Countries," International Food Policy Research Institute Discussion Paper 01029, Oct 2010; *World Livestock 2011.* UN FAO, 2011, p. 66.
28. Tim Lang, "From 'Value for Money' to 'Values for Money'? Ethical Food and Policy in Europe," *Enviro and Planning* A 42(8) 1814–1832, 2010.
29. "Pay the Price: An International Campaign to Raise the Price of Food," *The Ecologist*, Aug 5, 2010. facebook.com/pages/Pay-the-price, Mar 3, 2012.
30. Robert F. Kennedy Jr., "From Farms to Factories," in *The CAFO Reader.* D. Imhoff, ed., 2010, p. 205.
31. Barton Seaver, *For Cod and Country.* NY: Sterling, 2011.

32. Jennifer Jacquet and Daniel Pauly, "Seafood Stewardship in Crisis," *Nature* 467 (2) Sept 2010.

33. John Volpe et al., "How Green Is Your Eco-Label? Comparing the Environmental Benefits of Marine Aquaculture Standards," University of Victoria Seafood Ecology Research Group, Dec 2011.

34. SeaChoice eco-label, part of the Conservation Alliance for Seafood Solutions, seachoice.org, accessed Mar 8, 2012.

35. Nancy Kwon, "Get Hooked on Sustainable Seafood," *Canadian Grocer*, Sept 28, 2011; Hooked website, hookedinc.ca.

36. World Wildlife Fund, wwf.ca, accessed Mar 8, 2012.

37. Sustainable Table, "Eggs," sustainabletable.org, accessed Feb 2012.

38. Thanks to my family physician, Dr. Raymond McConville, for this wise reminder.

39. Vesanto Melina and Brenda Davis, *Becoming Vegetarian*. Wiley and Sons, 2003; Brenda Davis and Vesanto Melina, *Becoming Vegan*. Book Publishing Co., 2000; Marion Nestle. *What to Eat.* 2006.

40. Mark Bittman, *Food Matters*. 2009, p. 85.

41. Pimentel and Pimentel, "Sustainability of Meat-Based and Plant-Based Diets and the Environment," *Am J Clin Nutr* 78:3 (suppl) 660S–663S, 2003, p. 661S.

42. *World Livestock 2011: Livestock in Food Security*. UN FAO. "Safe" here is not just a minimum, but an average protein requirement for individuals, plus twice the standard deviation. It is, therefore, plenty for most people, p. 8–9.

43. Nestle, *What to Eat*. 2006, p. 73.

44. USDA Center for Nutrition Policy and Promotion dietary guidelines, "Pyramid Servings: How Much? How Many?" fns.usda.gov, 2010; "Choose My Plate," U.S. Dept of Agriculture, choosemyplate.gov; *Healthy Planet Eating: How Lower Meat Diets Can Save Lives and the Planet*. Friends of the Earth, 2010.

45. Canada's Food Guide, hc-sc.gc.ca, accessed Feb 22, 2012.

46. Melina and Davis, *Becoming Vegetarian*. Wiley, 2003, p. 80.

47. Craig and Marc Kielburger, "Can't Go the Whole Hog? Try Being a Flexivore," *Globe and Mail*, Oct 11, 2011, p. L3.

48. Paul Hawken, *Blessed Unrest: How the Largest Movement in the World Came into Being and Why No One Saw It Coming*. New York: Viking, 2007; Another excellent book is John Izzo's *Stepping Up: How Taking Responsibility Changes Everything*. San Francisco: Berrett-Koehler, 2012.

Chapter 8

1. Hans Schreier, Professor, Institute for Resources, Environment and Sustainability, University of British Columbia, personal interviews, 2011 and 2012.

2. Hans Schreier, "Agricultural Water Policy Challenges for BC," *Policy Options*, Jul–Aug 2009.

3. Hans Schreier, "Agriculture and Water: Harvesting Water Before Harvesting the Crop," Speaking of Science Lecture Series, Simon Fraser University, Vancouver, B.C., Oct 17, 2002.

4. Stefan Wirsenius and Fredrik Hedenus, "Policy Strategies for a Sustainable Food System: Options for Protecting the Climate," in D'Silva and Webster, eds., 2010, p. 246.
5. Corinna Hawkes, "Food Taxes: What Type of Evidence Is Available to Inform Policy Development?" *Nutrition Bulletin* 37: 51–56, 2012.
6. Mark Bittman, "Bad Food? Tax It, and Subsidize Vegetables," *New York Times*, Jul 24, 2011.
7. "Denmark Introduces World's First Food Fat Tax," BBC News Europe, bbc.co .uk, Oct 1, 2011, accessed Mar 7, 2012.
8. Peter Singer, "Make Meat-Eaters Pay: Ethicist Proposes Radical Tax, Says They're Killing Themselves and the Planet," *NY Daily News*, Oct 25, 2009; Nathan Fiala, "The Greenhouse Hamburger," *Scientific American*, Feb 2009. In his blogs, Dr. Fiala has called for meat taxes, or at least an end to high U.S. subsidies for meat production. Food writer Mark Bittman has called for more taxes on junk and processed foods: "Bad Food? Tax It, and Subsidize Vegetables," *New York Times*, Jul 23, 2011.
9. Hawkes, 2012, p. 51.
10. Organization for Economic Cooperation and Development, "Promoting Sustainable Consumption: Good Practices in OECD Countries," 2008, p. 13.
11. A. M. Thow, et al., "The Effect of Fiscal Policy on Diet, Obesity and Chronic Disease: A Systematic Review," *Bulletin World Health Organization* 88: 609–614, 2010.
12. *World Livestock 2011: Livestock in Food Security.* UN FAO, 2011, p. 66; As well, surveys conducted in Canada in 2009 and 2010, by Harris/Decima for the Vancouver Humane Society, showed that more than 70% of Canadians say they would pay extra for animal products that are certified humane.
13. Anthony McMichael and Ainslie Butler, "Environmentally Sustainable and Equitable Meat Consumption in a Climate Change World," in D'Silva and Webster, eds., 2010, p. 186.
14. Jonathon Porritt, "Confronting Policy Dilemmas," in D'Silva and Webster, eds., p. 275–286, 2010, p. 285.
15. Porritt, 2010, p. 275.
16. Jane Fearnley-Whittingstall, *The Ministry of Food: Thrifty Wartime Ways to Feed Your Family Today.* London: Hodder & Stoughton and the Imperial War Museum, 2010.
17. Tony Judt, *Postwar: A History of Europe Since 1945.* Penguin, 2005, p. 163.
18. Eleanor Boyle, "Could We Learn from the Ministry of Food?" eleanorboyle .com, Jul 8, 2010.
19. Porritt, 2010, p. 285.
20. Steinfeld et al., 2006, p. 222.
21. Tim Lang, Michelle Wu, and Martin Caraher, "Meat and Policy: Charting a Course Through the Complexity," in D'Silva and Webster, eds., 2010, p. 254.
22. *Vision Green 2011.* Outlines ideas for a national agricultural and food policy. Ottawa, Ontario: Green Party of Canada; Alex Atamanenko, *Food for Thought: Towards a National Food Strategy.* Ottawa: New Democratic Party of Canada,

2010; Michael Ignatieff, *Rural Canada Matters: Highlights of the Liberal Plan for Canada's First National Food Policy.* Ottawa: Liberal Party of Canada, 2010.

23. Canadian Federation of Agriculture, "Toward a National Food Strategy: Securing the Future of Food." Ottawa, Ontario, 2011; Canadian Agri-Food Policy Institute, "Canada's Agri-Food Destination: A New Strategic Approach." Ottawa, Ontario, 2011.

24. "Resetting the Table: A People's Food Policy for Canada," 2011, peoplesfoodpolicy.ca, accessed Mar 3, 2012.

25. Rod MacRae, "A Joined-Up Food Policy for Canada," *J Hunger and Environ Nutrition* 6(4) 424–457, 2011.

26. David Barling, Tim Lang, and Martin Caraher, "Joined-Up Food Policy? The Trials of Governance, Public Policy and the Food System," *Soc Policy Adm* 36: 556–574, 2002.

27. Rod MacRae, 2010, personal interview with author, November 24, 2010.

28. Lang, Barling, and Caraher, *Food Policy.* 2009.

29. Many analysts say industry plays a strong role in shaping de facto food policy. See Lang, Barling, and Caraher, 2009; Tim Lang and Michael Heasman, *Food Wars: The Global Battle for Mouths, Minds and Markets.* Earthscan, 2004; Marion Nestle, *Food Politics.* University of California Press, 2002.

30. Rod MacRae et al., *How Governments in Other Jurisdictions Successfully Support the Development of Organic Food and Farming.* organicagcentre.ca, 2004, p. 4–5, accessed Mar 3, 2012.

31. *The Farming Systems Trial.* Rodale Institute: Kutztown, PA, 2011, p. 4.

32. Centers for Disease Control, "Investigation Update: Multistate Outbreak of Human *Salmonella* Enteritidis Infections Associated with Shell Eggs," cdc.gov, updated Dec 2, 2010; "Wright County Egg Expands Nationwide Voluntary Recall of Shell Eggs Because of Possible Health Risk," FDA, Aug 18, 2010, fda.gov, accessed Mar 3, 2012

33. "Lessons Learned: Public Health Agency of Canada Response to the 2008 Listeriosis Outbreak: Executive Summary," hc-sc.gc.ca, p. 1, accessed Mar 8, 2012.

34. Sheila Weatherhill, independent investigator, "Listeriosis Investigative Review," notes for a news conference, Jul 21, 2009. listeriosis-listeriose.investigation-enquete.gc.ca.

35. Government of Canada, "What Led to the Outbreak?" listeriosis-listeriose.investigation-enquete.gc.ca, modified Jul 23, 2009.

36. Rachel Nowak, "Burp Vaccine Cuts Greenhouse Gas Emissions," *New Scientist*, Sept 25, 2004.

37. Council for Biotechnology Information, whybiotech.com, Mar 9, 2012.

38. Enviropig, uoguelph.ca, Mar 3, 2012.

39. AquaBounty, aquabounty.com, Mar 3, 2012.

40. Canadian Biotechnology Action Network, cban.ca.

41. "How 'Ya Gonna Keep 'Em Down on the Farm (After They've Seen Paree)?" was a popular song after WWI written by Joe Young and Sam M. Lewis with music by Walter Donaldson; it was published in 1918, and performed by many artists in the post-war years.

42. Healthy Food Action October e-news, "Ask Your U.S. Representative to Co-sponsor the Beginning Farmer and Rancher Opportunity Act of 2011," Oct 4, 2011.
43. farmstart.ca, accessed Mar 9, 2012; Daniel Imhoff, *Food Fight: The Citizen's Guide to the Next Food and Farm Bill.* Watershed Media, 2012, p. 92–93.
44. Bill McKibben, *Eaarth: Making a Life on a Tough New Planet.* St. Martin's Griffin, 2010, p. 174.
45. Rod MacRae, interview with author, Toronto, November, 2010.
46. For details on these and other organizations, see Appendix II.
47. Mark Bittman, "Bad Food? Tax It, and Subsidize Vegetables," *New York Times,* Jul 23, 2011.
48. Ibid.
49. Nicolette Hahn Niman, *Righteous Porkchop: Finding a Life and Good Food Beyond Factory Farms.* 2009; Niman Ranch, nimanranch.com, accessed Mar 9, 2012.
50. Good Shepherd Poultry Ranch, goodshepherdpoultryranch.com, accessed Mar 9, 2012.
51. Frank Reese Jr., owner of Good Shepherd Poultry, e-mail to author, January, 2012.
52. Michael McFadden of Farm Forward, e-mail to author, January, 2012.
53. Adele Hayes, e-mail to author, October, 2011.
54. Shannon Hayes, *The Grassfed Gourmet Cookbook: Healthy Cooking and Good Living with Pasture-Raised Foods.* Eating Fresh Publications, 2004.
55. Ronnie Cummins of the Organic Consumers Association (OCA), e-mail to author, October 25, 2011. There are probably 10,000 producers in the United States of organic (certified organic or not) animal products. There are about 25,000 certified organic farms and ranches in the United States, and many more that are not USDA certified as organic. Less than 5% of North American meat, dairy, and eggs are currently "organic"—either certified as such or using organic practices.
56. Bellarby et al., 2008; Steinfeld et al., 2006; Robert Goodland and Jeff Anhang, "Livestock and Climate Change: What If the Key Actors in Climate Change Are…Cows, Pigs, and Chickens?" *World Watch Magazine* Nov/Dec 2009, p. 10–19; B. P. Weidema et al., *Environmental Improvement Potentials of Meat and Dairy Products.* European Commission Joint Research Centre, 2008.
57. Steinfeld et al., 2006.
58. Manitoba Pork Council, *Embracing a Sustainable Future.* 2011.
59. "Sustainability at Tyson Foods: A Message from Our Chief Environmental Health and Safety Officer," tysonfoods.com, accessed Feb 19, 2012.
60. Lang, Barling, and Caraher, *Food Policy.* 2009; Steinfeld et al., 2006; Andrew Nikiforuk, "Factory Farming Is Polluting the Water Supply," in *Current Controversies: Pollution,* James Haley, ed. Greenhaven Press, 2003.
61. Problematic externalities have been extensively documented. See Steinfeld et al., 2006; Daniel Imhoff, *Food Fight.* 2012; and Doug Gurian-Sherman, *CAFOs Uncovered.* 2008.

62. Jules Pretty et al., "Policy Challenges and Priorities for Internalizing the Externalities of Modern Agriculture," *J Enviro Planning Management* 44(2) 263–283, 2001; James Merchant, "Advancing Industrial Livestock Production: Health Effects Research and Sustainability," *Epidemiology* 22(2) 216–218, 2011.

63. Steinfeld et al., 2006, p. 223; Henning Steinfeld and Pierre Gerber, "Livestock Production and the Global Environment: Consume Less or Produce Better?" *PNAS* 107(43) 18237–8, 2010, p. 18238; Steinfeld, Gerber, and Opio, "Responses on Environmental Issues," in *Livestock in a Changing Landscape*. Steinfeld et al., Island Press, 2010.

64. Imhoff, 2007; Gurian-Sherman, 2008.

65. McKibben, 2010, p. 177.

66. Gary Williams, Professor of Agricultural Economics, Texas A&M University, speaking at "Reforming the 2012 Farm Bill," forum at the Harvard School of Public Health, Oct 20, 2011, hsph.harvard.edu, accessed Jan, 2012.

67. Steinfeld et al., 2006, p. 232.

68. Council on Foreign Relations, "Should the U.S. Cut Its Farm Subsidies?" cfr.org, 2007.

69. Elanor Starmer and Timothy Wise, *Feeding at the Trough: Industrial Livestock Firms Saved $35 Billion from Low Feed Prices*. Global Development and Environment Institute, Tufts University, Policy Brief no. 07–03, Dec 2007.

70. Gurian-Sherman, 2008.

71. Daniel Imhoff, *Food Fight*. 2012, p. 13.

72. *Citizens' Guide to Confronting a Factory Farm*. Saskatoon, SK: Beyond Factory Farming Coalition, 2007, p. 8.2.

73. Thomas Pawlick, *The War in the Country*. Vancouver: Greystone, 2009, p. 10.

74. Brigitt Johnson, "Impact of the Meat Inspection Regulation on Slaughter Capacity in the North Okanagan Regional District: Final Report," sponsored by the North Okanagan Food Action Coalition, Jan 2008.

75. Rod MacRae, interview with author, November, 2010.

76. Ibid.

77. Fred Tait, "Pork, Politics and Power," in Ervin et al., *Beyond Factory Farming*. 2003, p. 39–58.

78. Nicole Fadellin and Michael Broadway, "Canada's Prairies: From Breadbasket to Feed Bunker and Hog Trough," *Geography* 91(1) 84–88, 2006.

79. David Kirby, *Animal Factory*. St. Martin's Press, 2010.

80. Daniel Imhoff, 2012, p. 60–61; Gurian-Sherman, 2008, p. 29.

81. Gurian-Sherman, 2008, p. 29.

82. Pawlick, 2009, p. 108.

83. agcanada.com, accessed Mar 3, 2012.

84. "Letter to President Barack Obama," Robert Martin, Senior Officer, Pew Environment Group, Pew Commission, Aug 31, 2009.

85. David Molden, ed., *Water for Food, Water for Life: A Comprehensive Assessment of Water Management in Agriculture*. International Water Management Institute, London: Earthscan, 2007.

86. Steinfeld et al., 2006, p. 230.

87. "Environmental Coalition Calls for Full Cost Pricing of Water," environment
.probeinternational.org, Sept 1, 2009, accessed Feb 2012.

88. Molden, ed., *Water for Food, Water for Life.* 2007.

89. The PigSite, "Despite Moratorium, More Hog Farms Built in North Carolina
in Past 10 years," thepigsite.com, accessed Mar 23, 2007.

90. Ibid.

91. Food and Water Watch press release, "NC CAFO Moratorium Fails to Slow
Factory Farm Growth," locallygrownnews.com, Dec 2, 2010, accessed Mar 9,
2012.

92. Ibid. Also see *Factory Farm Nation.* 2010.

93. More on these organizations in Appendix II.

94. *Impacts of Antimicrobial Growth Promoter Termination in Denmark.* Denmark: World Health Organization, Nov 2002, p. 8.; Bonfoh et al., "Human
Health Hazards," in Steinfeld et al., 2010, p. 212.

95. Andrew Gunther, "The FDA Fails the Public on Antibiotics Once Again," huff
ingtonpost.com, Jan 9, 2012.

96. U.S. Federal Register, "FDA Notice on Antibiotics," gpo.gov, Dec 22, 2011.

97. Manitoba Pork Council, *Embracing a Sustainable Future.* Mar 2011, p. 38; Mike
Teillet, manager of sustainable development programs, Manitoba Pork Council, e-mail to author, December 7, 2011.

98. Jason Johnson, "Ides Transition Open Feedlot to Hoop Buildings," USDA
Conservation Showcase, Aug 2011; Mark Honeyman et al., "Managing Market
Pigs in Hoop Structures," Extension 2010, extension.org.

99. Humane Society of the U.S., "HSUS and Egg Industry Agree to Promote Federal Standards for Hens," humanesociety.org, Mar 9, 2012.

100. Humane Society of the U.S., "California Enacts Landmark Bill Banning Tail
Docking of Cows," press release, Oct 12, 2009.

101. Michigan Policy Network, "Michigan Governor Signs Law Giving Farm Animals Room," michiganpolicy.com, accessed Mar 8.

102. Ann Clark, "The Future Is Organic: But It's More Than Organic," *Energy Bulletin*, Jan 14, 2010, p. 10.

103. Seth Joel, Seth Joel Photography, Los Angeles, CA.

104. Compassion in World Farming, "Global Warming: Climate Change and Farm
Animal Welfare: Summary Report," 2008.

105. Farm Animal Welfare Awards, "The Fate of Billions of Animals Is in Our
Hands," Compassion in World Farming, ciwf.org.uk, accessed Mar 11, 2012.

106. Joyce D'Silva, Compassion in World Farming, e-mail to author, January 4,
2012.

107. *Livestock's Long Shadow.* 2006; UN FAO, *World Livestock 2011.* 2011.

108. Pete Smith et al., "Agriculture," in *Climate Change 2007: Mitigation. Contribution of Working Group III to the Fourth Assessment Report of the Intergovernmental Panel on Climate Change.* Cambridge University Press, 2007.

109. C. Nellemann et al., eds., "The Environmental Food Crisis." UN Environmental Program, 2009, unep.org, Dec, 2011.

110. McMichael et al., 2007.
111. McMichael and Butler, 2010, p. 185.

Chapter 9

1. Sidney Mintz, *Tasting Food, Tasting Freedom: Excursions into Eating, Culture, and the Past.* Boston: Beacon Press, 1996; Martin Caraher, Heidi Baker, and Maureen Burns, "Children's Views of Cooking and Food Preparation," *British Food Journal* 106 (4) 255–273, 2004.
2. Many researchers have demonstrated the superiority of low-meat diets for health, e.g., Marion Nestle, *What to Eat.* 2006, p. 146; Barry Popkin, *The World Is Fat.* 2009; and T. Colin Campbell, *The China Study.* 2006.
3. Carol Adams, *The Sexual Politics of Meat: A Feminist-Vegetarian Critical Theory.* First published 1990. Republished by NY: Continuum, 2000.
4. McDonald's television ad, voice-over says: "It makes men act like men," Jan 2012.
5. Erik De Bakker and Hans Dagevos, "Reducing Meat Consumption in Today's Consumer Society: Questioning the Citizen-Consumer Gap," *J Agric Enviro Ethics* 1–18, Sept 25, 2011, p. 5.
6. Project CHEF, projectchef.ca, Mar 9, 2012.
7. Barb Finley, chef at Project CHEF, e-mail to author, Nov, 2011.
8. Bill Moyer, *Doing Democracy: The MAP Model for Organizing Social Movements.* Gabriola Island, B.C.: New Society Publishers, 2001, p. 44–45.
9. Bill Moyer, 2001, p. 181.
10. Malcolm Gladwell, *The Tipping Point: How Little Things Can Make a Big Difference.* Little, Brown, 2000.
11. The National Conference to End Factory Farming: For Health, Environment, and Farm Animals. Held in Arlington, VA, Oct 27–29, 2011. Organized by Farm Sanctuary, a non-governmental organization that rescues abused farm animals, educates, and advocates for change to the ways we treat animals.
12. Susie Coston, Farm Sanctuary national director, told the story of Rosie the pig.
13. John Ikerd, professor emeritus of agricultural economics, University of Missouri, speaking at the National Conference to End Factory Farming, 2011.
14. Ikerd conference speech, 2011.
15. Ibid.
16. Steinfeld et al., 2006, p. 222.
17. Tim Lang, Michelle Wu and Martin Caraher, in D'Silva and Webster, eds., 2010, p. 256. Dr. Lang is head of the Centre for Food Policy, City University, London, England.
18. Lang et al., in D'Silva and Webster, eds., 2010, p. 256.
19. Peter Rosset, *Food Is Different: Why We Must Get the WTO Out of Agriculture.* Fernwood Publishing, 2006; Raj Patel, *Stuffed and Starved: The Hidden Battle for the World Food System.* Melville House, 2007.
20. Olivier de Schutter, UN Special Rapporteur on the Right to Food, "The World Trade Organization and the Post-Global Food Crisis Agenda," Activity Report,

Nov, 2011; "Lamy and UN Rights Expert in Row over Food Security," Third World Network Info Service, Dec 21, 2011, twnside.org.

21. Clean Environment Commission of Manitoba, "Environmental Sustainability and Hog Production in Manitoba," Dec 2007, p. 46.
22. "The Perils of Poultry," *Canad Medical Assn J* 181(1–2) 2009.
23. Joel Novek, "Intensive Livestock Operations, Disembedding, and Community Polarization in Manitoba," *Soc Nat Res* 16: 567–581, 2003, p. 567.
24. Marion Nestle, *What to Eat.* 2006, p. 149.
25. "Environmental Sustainability and Hog Production in Manitoba," 2007, p. vii.
26. Lang et al., *Food Policy.* 2009, p. 130.
27. Tim Lang and Geoff Rayner, "Overcoming Policy Cacophony on Obesity: An Ecological Public Health Framework for Policymakers," *Obesity Reviews* 8(S1) 165–181, 2007.
28. Elizabeth Brubaker, *Greener Pastures: Decentralizing the Regulation of Agricultural Pollution.* University of Toronto Press, 2007.
29. David Kirby, *Animal Factory.* St. Martin's Press, 2010.
30. Organization of Economic Cooperation and Development (OECD), *Divided We Stand: Why Inequality Keeps Rising.* Dec 2011.
31. Wenonah Hauter, Executive Director, Food and Water Watch, speaking at the National Conference to End Factory Farming, 2011.
32. U.S. Dept of Justice, Agriculture and Antitust Enforcement Issues in Our 21st Century Economy," justice.gov, accessed Feb 2012; Food First, "Food Sovereignty Alliance Activists Submit 240,000 Petitions Demanding Action to Curb Food Monopolies," foodfirst.org, Dec 6, 2010.
33. Steinfeld et al., 2006, p. 222.
34. Animal Agriculture Alliance, soundagscience.org.
35. Animal Agriculture Alliance, Stakeholders Summit, May 5–6, 2011. Session: Insider Threats: Strategies for Mitigation, eventfarm.com, accessed Feb 14, 2012.
36. Canadian Meat Council Strategies. Lobbying Activity Information, cmc-cvc.com, accessed Feb 11, 2012. Under "Lobbying Activity Information," the site said the Council will "advocate for an amendment to the (Food and Drugs) Act to allow for the immediate approval in Canada of all antimicrobial agents currently approved by European Union and by the U.S. Food and Drugs Administration."
37. Jonathon Porritt, "Confronting Policy Dilemmas," in D'Silva and Webster, 2010, p. 277.
38. Marion Nestle, *Food Politics.* University of California Press, 2002, p. 40.
39. Ibid., p. 40–42.
40. Ibid., p. 78.
41. Justin Bekelman, Yan Li, and Cary Gross, "Scope and Impact of Financial Conflicts of Interest in Biomedical Research," *JAMA* 289(4) 454–465, 2003, p. 459.
42. Marion Nestle, "Big Food, Big Agra, and the Research University," *Academe*, Nov–Dec 2010, p. 47–49, p. 48.

43. Robert Martin, "Putting Meat on the Table: Industrial Farm Animal Production in America," Pew Commission, 2008, p. viii.
44. Ibid.
45. Rick Dove, volunteer with Neuse Riverkeeper organization, personal interview in North Carolina, July 2011.
46. "Pork is considered a red meat," according to CFIA (Canadian Food Inspection Agency). E-mail to author, April 27, 2011.
47. National Pork Board, 1987 advertising campaign, porkbeinspired.com.
48. Cattlemen's Beef Board and National Cattlemen's Beef Association, beefits whatsfordinner.com.
49. Meat and Livestock Australia, 2006, acutabove.net.au.
50. Nestle, *What to Eat.* p. 142.
51. USDA Research and Promotion Programs, ams.usda.gov; David Shipman, "Industry Insight: Checkoff Programs Empower Business," USDA blog, Sept 21, 2011, blogs.usda.gov.
52. Beef Board, beefboard.org.
53. Pork Checkoff, pork.org.
54. Nestle, *What to Eat.* p. 141.
55. Manitoba Pork Council, manitobapork.com, accessed Feb 11, 2012.
56. Dairy Council of California, dairycouncilofca.org, accessed Feb 11, 2012.
57. Wayne Pacelle, speech at the National Conference to End Factory Farming, 2011.
58. Steinfeld et al., 2006, p. 221.
59. Chef Laura Lee, Napa Valley Cooking School, e-mail to the author, July, 2011.
60. Rod MacRae, et al., *How Governments in Other Jurisdictions Successfully Support the Development of Organic Food and Farming.* Written with financial support from Agriculture and AgriFood Canada and the Laidlaw Foundation, Feb 9, 2004, p. 1–59, p. 8.
61. Fred Tait, "Pork, Politics, and Power," in Ervin et al., *Beyond Factory Farming.* CCPA, 2003, p. 39–58.
62. Ibid., p. 50.
63. Ibid., p. 49.
64. Ibid., p. 50.
65. NFU, "National Farmers' Union Submission to Govt of Manitoba," Saskatoon, SK, Apr 15, 2004, p. 11–12.
66. Roger Epp, "Beyond Our Own Backyards: Factory Farming and the Political Economy of Extraction," in Ervin et al., eds., *Beyond Factory Farming.* p. 179–180. Dr. Epp is a professor of political science at the University of Alberta.
67. Ibid.

Chapter 10

1. The operation is Waratah Downs Organic Farm near Ottawa, Ontario, which I visited in the fall of 2010.
2. Sap Bush Hollow Farm, sapbush.com, accessed Mar 3, 2012.
3. Greenling local organic food delivery, greenling.com, accessed, Mar 3, 2012.

4. Website of greenling.com and personal e-mail communication from the company,
5. *Super Size Me.* Documentary film by Morgan Spurlock exploring fast food, 2004.
6. *Food Inc.* Documentary film about America's corporate food industry. Oscar-nominated and widely watched, 2008.
7. Thank you to Conner Ingram, his mother Linda Watt, and his brother Miles Ingram. My appreciation to the Vancouver Humane Society that profiled Conner and Miles in their fall 2011 newsletter, vancouverhumanesociety.bc.ca.

Appendix I

1. ted.com/talks/graham_hill_weekday_vegetarian.html. Accessed March 4, 2012.
2. Greens in San Francisco, introduced at the start of Chapter 7, is one such vegetarian restaurant. Others include Toronto's Fresh, Seattle's Café Flora, and San Francisco's Millennium. In New York City, there are many choices, including Candle Café, Candle 79, Zen Palate, and Blossom. If you're in London, there's Tibits, Chutney's, Mildred's, and many others.

Index

Treacy, Dennis, 108–109
Tyedmers, Peter, 102

U
UN Environmental Program (UNEP), 156
UN Food and Agriculture Organization (FAO), 5, 15, 28–29, 30, 37–38, 52, 55–56, 87, 128, 156, 162, 166–167, 170
United Nations, 19, 87
University of California at Davis, 30
US Centers for Disease Control, 71, 76
US Department of Agriculture, 16, 165
US Department of Justice, 166
US Farm Bill, 103–104, 148
US Food and Drug Administration (FDA), 58, 63–64, 69, 152–153

V
values, and food systems, 94–96, 107
Vancouver Humane Society, 95
Vandana, Shiva, 120
vegetables, 121–130, 181–194. *See also* plant foods.
vegetarian diet, 9–10, 72–73, 101, 115, 121, 127, 181–194
Vesanto, Melina, 130
Vision for Fair Food and Farming, 39–40

W
Walkerton, Ontario, 46–47
wastage, of animal-source food, 122

waste. *See* human sewage; manure.
Waterkeeper Alliance, 41, 44
water
  and agriculture, 54–56, 146
  pricing of, 151
  quality of, 41–56, 81
  shortages of, 54–55, 151
Water for Food, Water for Life, 151
Webb, Don, 7, 45–46, 94–96
Weekday Vegetarian, 115, 181
Weida, William, 83
Whole Foods, 124
Williams, Gary, 147
Williams, Mike, 48–49, 107–108, 150
Winfrey, Oprah, 22
Wing, Steve, 82
Wirsenius, Stefan, 133
Wise, Timothy 147–148
World Cancer Research Fund, 75–76, 77, 114
World Health Organization, 61, 67–68, 69, 91, 152
World Trade Organization (WTO), 105–106, 163
World Wildlife Fund Canada, 126
Wu, Michelle, 163

Y
Yale University, 168

Z
zoonoses, 59–63

About the Author

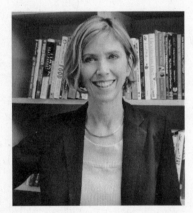

ELEANOR BOYLE is an educator and writer who focuses on how we can make our food systems and meal choices sustainable, healthy, and compassionate. She teaches, facilitates community discussions, and writes, to educate consumers and to work for better food policy. Eleanor has an honors BA in Behavioral Sciences from the University of Chicago, a PhD in Neuroscience from the University of British Columbia, and an MSc in Food Policy from City University in London. She has been asked to speak at numerous conferences on food issues. Eleanor has worked for newspapers and television, studied at Cambridge University on a press fellowship, and worked in Africa as a UN consultant to journalists. A long-time college teacher, she co-wrote a book with her husband, Harley Rothstein, on how to be an effective university instructor. They live in Vancouver where Eleanor keeps fit, enjoys spending time with family, and is an enthusiastic cook. You can read her website and blog at eleanorboyle.com, and on the High Steaks site at highsteaksbook.com.

If you have enjoyed *High Steaks,* you might also enjoy other

BOOKS TO BUILD A NEW SOCIETY

Our books provide positive solutions for people who want to
make a difference. We specialize in:

**Sustainable Living • Green Building • Peak Oil
Renewable Energy • Environment & Economy
Natural Building & Appropriate Technology
Progressive Leadership • Resistance and Community
Educational & Parenting Resources**

For a full list of NSP's titles, please call 1-800-567-6772 *or check out our website* at:

www.newsociety.com

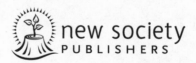